Identification and Management of Antiparasitic Resistance

The Editors

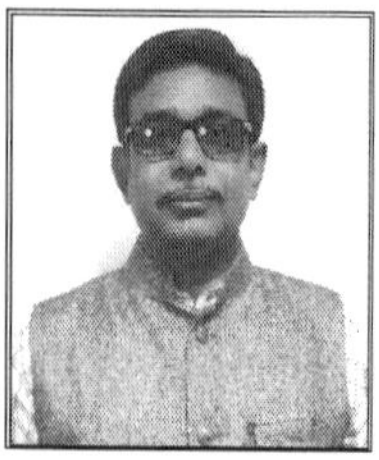

Dr. Giridhari Das, Professor and Head, Department of Veterinary Parasitology, College of Vety. Sci. and AH., Nanaji Deshmukh Veterinary Science University, Jabalpur also working as Controller of Examination of this University. Dr. Das was a graduate of West Bengal University of Animal and Fishery Sciences, Kolkata and in pursuance to his higher studies he got admitted in IVRI, Izatnagar with ICAR-JRF and in continuation completed his doctoral degree with ICAR-SRF in Veterinary Parasitology. Dr Das is having more than 21 years of teaching and research experience in different capacity and guided more than 25 master's and doctoral students as major and minor advisor. Dr. Das is the recipient of National Scholarship, Dr. V.S. Alwar Award of Indian Association for the Advancement of Veterinary Parasitology (IAAVP) twice in the year 2003 and 2017. He has published several review articles, book chapters, manuals and more than 80 research papers in national and international journals of reputes.

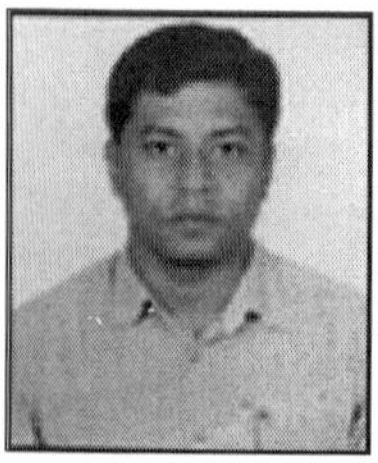

Dr. Suman Kumar was awarded B. V. Sc. and A. H. degree by University of Agricultural Sciences (UAS), Dharwad, Karnataka, in the year 2002. He did his M. V. Sc. and Ph.D. degree from Rajendra Agricultural University (RAU), Pusa, Bihar, in the years 2006 and 2010, respectively in the discipline of Veterinary Parasitology. He started his academic carrier as Assistant Professor, Department of Veterinary Parasitology, College of Veterinary Science and A. H., NDVSU, Rewa. Presently, he is serving as Assistant Professor at College of Veterinary Science and A.H., Nanaji Deshmukh Veterinary Science University, Jabalpur, Madhya Pradesh. He has more than 10 years of teaching and research experience. He has published several book chapters, manuals and more than 35 research papers in national and international journals of reputes.

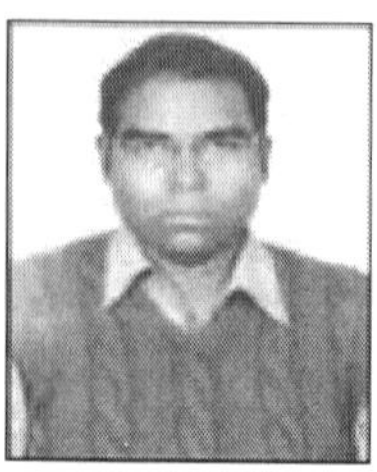

Dr. Subhradal Nath is presently working as Assistant Professor at College of Veterinary Science and A. H., Nanaji Deshmukh Veterinary Science University, Jabalpur, Madhya Pradesh. He did his M. V. Sc. and Ph.D. degree from IGKV, Raipur (C.G.) and CGKV, Durg (C.G.) in the years 2008 and 2019, respectively in the discipline of Veterinary Parasitology. Dr. Nath has an experience of more than 10 years in the field of teaching and research. He has published two books and more than 35 articles in various journals of national and international repute. He has received many awards and honours and is a recipient of Rashtrapati Scout by His Excellency, Honourable President of India in the year 1999.

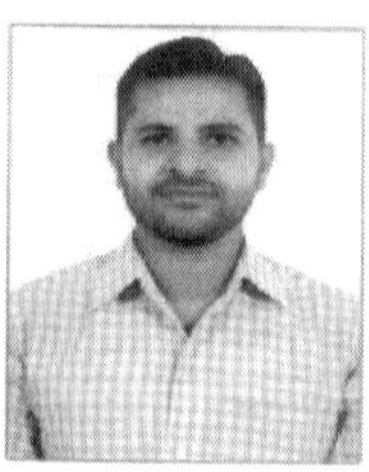

Dr. Rupesh Verma completed his B.V.Sc. and A.H. degree from the College of Veterinary Science and A.H., Mhow, (MP) in 2014, and his M.V.Sc. degree in Veterinary Parasitology from the IVRI, Bareilly (UP). He worked as Veterinary Assistant Surgeon for two years at Mandsaur, Department of Animal Husbandry and Dairying, Madhya Pradesh. Presently, he is working as Assistant Professor in the Department of Veterinary Parasitology, COVSc and AH., NDVSU, Jabalpur (MP). He has authored one book, 5 book chapter and more than 25 research papers in national and international journals.

Identification and Management of Antiparasitic Resistance

— *Editors* —

Dr. Giridhari Das

Dr. Suman Kumar

Dr. Subhradal Nath

Dr. Rupesh Verma

ASTRAL

Publishing Authors Across the Globe

2025

Daya Publishing House®

A Division of

Astral International Pvt. Ltd.

New Delhi – 110 002

ISBN: 978-93-5919-207-9

Published by : **Daya Publishing House®**
A Division of
Astral International Pvt. Ltd.
– ISO 9001:2015 Certified Company –
4736/23, Ansari Road, Darya Ganj
New Delhi-110 002
Ph. 011-43549197
E-mail: info@astralint.com
Website: www.astralint.com

Printed at : **Replika Press Pvt Ltd**

Preface

Livestock rearing has grown in popularity in recent decades due to its lucrative economic prospects, especially when reared in an intensive and semi-intensive system. These farming systems significantly increase the risk of parasitic disease in animals, resulting in significant economic losses to farmers since the disease is mostly subclinical and most animals do not exhibit symptoms. There is no question that chemotherapy is an excellent remedy for a wide range of parasitic infections. Unfortunately, the emergence of antiparasitic drug resistance is jeopardizing the usefulness of available drugs. Although antiparasitic resistance in animals does not directly affect human health, but it poses a significant threat to animal health and can lead to production losses in food-producing species.

The numerous reports emphasize the urgent need to redouble efforts to combat drug resistance and outlines immediate policymaker actions that would aid in optimizing animal health production. These include judicial use of existing antiparasitic drugs; using alternatives such as herbal, biological, genetic and immunological; enhancing efforts to monitor and control infections and increasing funding for the development of new drugs. Identifying and diagnosing resistance status will be vital for future parasite control programme. Modern molecular techniques may be able to meet the demand for early and accurate drug resistance detection in a variety of parasitic species.

The book is a compilation of information regarding advancement in the field of detection of anthelmintic, acaricidal and antiprotozoal drug resistance and their mitigation strategies, as well as hands-on-training to diagnose the same. This book will be a milestone for students, faculty and researcher who want to carry out research in similar areas.

Editor of this book are highly thankful to all the authors who contributed their valuable research works.

Dr. Giridhari Das

Dr. Suman Kumar

Dr. Subhradal Nath

Dr. Rupesh Verma

Contents

Chapter 1

Status of Anthelmintic Resistance in India

M. Sankar, K. A. Yashica, V.K, Tiwari, V. Prasanth, M. Silamparasan, R. Garg and S. Ghosh

Indian Veterinary Research Institute, Izatnagar – 243 122, Uttar Pradesh

Introduction

Anthelmintic resistance (AR) is a pre adaptive phenomenon occurs in a helminth population as a rare allele and is heritable. When selection pressure take place due to anthelmintic treatment, the rare allele loss the sensitivity of anthelmintics but sensitive parasite dies due to drug effect. These heritable changes include genetic and epigenetic change. Genetic changes are mutations, deletions or amplifications of specific genes and epigenetic changes whereby methylation of genes or promoter regions of the genes change the gene expression in response to the drug (Fojo, 2007). According to World Association for the Advancement of Veterinary Parasitology (WAAVP), anthelmintic resistance is the failure of a drug to reduce faecal nematode egg count by at least 95 per cent (Geary *et al.*, 2012). The rate at which anthelmintic resistance develops is based on the number of genes involved and whether they are dominant or recessive. Gene dominance refers to the ability of heterozygotes to survive a particular drug. If a drug kills the same high percentage of heterozygotes as the susceptible heterozygotes, the resistance gene is recessive. If the heterozygous genotype has equivalent ability to survive the resistant homozygote, the resistance gene is dominant. In India, the first anthelmintic resistance was reported from State Sheep and Wool Research Station, Pashulok, Rishikesh, Uttarakhand in *H. contortus* to phenothiazine and thiabendazole in sheep (Varshney and Singh, 1976).

Mechanism of Resistance of Anthelmintic Drugs

Various mechanisms are involved for drug resistance in helminths. Being higher eukaryotes, helminths adapt multiple strategies to evade drug effects through evolution. The major mechanism appears to be loss or decrease of the target site/receptor affinity to a drug. The P-glycoprotein (PGP), a multi-drug resistant cascade ion proteinis responsible for active transport of drugs (including ivermectin, benzimidazoles and imidazothiazole derivatives) from cytoplasm to outside cell which lead to multi-drug resistance. For BZ resistance, various studies proved single nucleotide 196 polymorphisms (SNP) at codons 167, 198 and 200 of the β-tubulin isotype 1, are responsible for resistance in helminths.

Status of Anthelmintic Resistance in India

In India, anthelmintic resistance in livestock has been reported from all the major states against commonly used anthelmintics such as benzimidazoles, levamisole, closantel and ivermectin in helminths of cattle, sheep, goat and equine. Most of the studies conducted includes FECRT, EHA and in few studies, assays such as Larval development assay, however, in recent years molecular assays like allele specific PCR, Restriction fragment length polymorphism (RFLP-PCR) are being employed.

Table 1.1: State-wise Report of AR for Various Drugs in Livestock in India by Conventional Methods

State	*Species*	*Drug*	*Reference*
Assam	Cattle	Benzimidazole, Levamisole	Choudhury *et al.*,2018; Choudhury and Bulbul, 2020
Andhra Pradesh	Sheep	Albendazole, Levamisole	Gill, 1996
Bihar	Goat	Fenbendazole, Levamisole, Ivermectin, Morantel	Kumar *et al.*, 2015
Chhattishgarh	Cattle	Albendazole, Levamisole, Ivermectin	Kumar *et al.*, 2014
	Goat	Albendazole, Levamisole, Ivermectin	Kumar *et al.*, 2014
	Goat	Albendazole	Rawte *et al.*, 2015
Gujarat	Sheep	Albendazole, Levamisole	Gill, 1996
	Sheep	Albendazole, Tetramisole, Ivermectin	Makvana *et al.*, 2009
	Goat	Albendazole, Levamisole, Ivermectin	Gelot *et al.*, 2016
Haryana	Sheep	Fenbendazole	Yadav *et al.*, 1990
	Sheep	Fenbendazole, Levamisole, Morantel	Yadav *et al.*, 1993

State	Species	Drug	Reference
	Goat	Fenbendazole, Levamisole, Thiophanate, Morantel	Uppal *et al.*, 1992
	Sheep	Fenbendazole	Kumar *et al.*, 1994
	Sheep	Fenbendazole	Uppal *et al.*, 1993
	Goat	Levamisole	Uppal *et al.*, 1993
	Goat	Fenbendazole, Levamisole, Morantel	Sing and Yadav, 1997
	Sheep	Fenbendazole, Levamisole, Morantel	Sing and Yadav, 1997
	Sheep	Fenbendazole, Levamisole, Morantel	Yadav *et al.*, 1995
	Cattle	Morantel	Yadav and verma, 1997
	Sheep	Closantel	Gupta *et al.*, 2003
	Goat	Fenbendazole, Morantel	Das and Singh, 2005
	Sheep	Fenbendazole, Rafoxanide, Morantel	Das and Singh, 2005
	Sheep	Fenbendazole, Tetramisole	Sangwan *et al.*, 2006
	Sheep	Fenbendazole, Tetramisole, Morantel	Chaudhri *et al.*, 2007
	Sheep	Morantel, Ivermectin	Singh and Gupta, 2010
	Sheep	Fenbendazole, Morantel	Das and Singh, 2010
	Goat	Fenbendazole	Das and Singh, 2010
	Goat	Ivermectin	Satyavir and Poonia, 2011
	Goat	Fenbendazole, Ivermectin	Priyanka *et al.*, 2013
	Cattle	Albendazole, Fenbendazole, levamisole	Sudharani *et al.*, 2013
	Sheep	Levamisole, Ivermectin	Singh *et al.*, 2015
	Sheep	Fenbendazole, Levamisole, Ivermectin	Ruchi *et al.*, 2015
	Sheep	Fenbendazole, Levamisole, MorantelIvermectin	Suresh and Satyavir, 2016
	Cattle	Fenbendazole	Singh, 2017
	Cattle	Albendazole	Sukhjeet and Satyavir, 2018
	Sheep	Fenbendazole, Morantel, Ivermectin	Priyanka *et al.*, 2019
	Goat	Fenbendazole, Ivermectin, Morantel	Priyanka *et al.*, 2019
	Goat	Fenbendazole, Morantel	Kalkal *et al.*, 2019, Vohra *et al.*, 2019
	Sheep	Fenbendazole, Morantel	Kalkal *et al.*, 2019, Vohra *et al.*, 2019
Jammu and Kashmir	Sheep	Tetramisole	Itoo*et al.*, 2012
	Sheep	Fenbendazole, Ivermectin	Shahardar *et al.*, 2014
	Goat	Fenbendazole	Sharma *et al.*, 2015

State	Species	Drug	Reference
	Goat	Albendazole, Fenbendazole	Bulbul *et al.*, 2018
	Sheep	Fenbendazole	Bulbul *et al.*, 2018
	Cattle	Fenbendazole, Ivermectin	Bulbul *et al.*, 2018
	Cattle	Closantel	Bushra *et al.*, 2019
	Goat	Fenbendazole, Ivermectin, Closantel	Bihaqi *et al.*, 2020
Karnataka	Sheep	Fenbendazole	Amulya *et al.*, 2016
		Fenbendazole, Ivermectin	Rathod *et al.*, 2017
	Sheep	Fenbendazole, Ivermectin	Veena *et al.*, 2020
Kerala	Goat	Albendazole, Ivermectin, Morantel	Deepa *et al.*, 2007
	Goat	Benzimidazole	Rajagopal *et al.*, 2013; 2017
Madhya Pradesh	Goat	Fenbendazole, Levamisole	Das *et al.*, 2015
	Goat	Fenbendazole	Dixit *et al.*, 2017
	Goat	Albendazole, Levamisole	Shakya *et al.*, 2018
Maharastra	Goat	Albendazole	Ghalsasi *et al.*, 2012
	Sheep	Albendazole	Ghalsasi *et al.*, 2012
Punjab	Sheep	Fenbendazole	Buttar *et al.*, 2011
	Sheep	Fenbendazole, Levamisole, MorantelIvermectin	Buttar *et al.*, 2012
	Goat	Fenbendazole, Ivermectin	Singh, 2012
	Goat	Fenbendazole	Singh *et al.*, 2017
	Sheep	Fenbendazole	Singh *et al.*, 2017
	Goat	Fenbendazole, Levamisole, Ivermectin	Pawar *et al.*, 2019
Rajasthan	Sheep	Levamisole, Albendazole	Gill,1996
	Sheep	Tetramisole, Rafoxanide, Fenbendazole	Swarnkar *et al.*, 1999
	Sheep	Tetramisole, Rafoxanide, Fenbendazole	Swarnkar *et al.*, 2001
	Sheep	Benzimidazolezimi	Maharshi *et al.*, 2011
	Goat	Fenbendazole, Levamisole	Godara*et al.*, 2011
	Sheep	Tetramisole, Benzimidazole	Swarnkar and Singh, 2012
	Goat	FenbendazoleLevamisole and Oxyclozanide	Lata, 2018
	Sheep	FenbendazoleLevamisole and Oxyclozanide	Lata, 2018
Tamil Nadu	Sheep	Albendazole, Levamisole	Gill, 1996
	Sheep	Tetramisole, Fenbendazole	Jeyathilakan *et al.*, 2003
	Sheep	Levamisole, Fenbendazole	Sundaram *et al.*, 2005
		Benzimidazole, Levamisole, Morantel, Ivermectin	Arunachalam *et al.*, 2005, 2013

State	Species	Drug	Reference
	Goat	Benzimidazole, Levamisole, Morantel, Ivermectin	Arunachalam *et al.*, 2013
	Sheep	Fenbendazole and Albendazole	Meenakshisundaram *et al.*, 2014
	Goat	Fenbendazole, Levamisole	Varadharajan and Vijayalakshmi, 2015; Manikkavasagan *et al.*, 2015
	Sheep	Fenbendazole, Tetramisole	Vijayasarathi *et al.*, 2016
	Sheep	Fenbendazole	Sahoo *et al.*, 2018
	Sheep	Levamisole, Fenbendazole	Varadharajan *et al.*, 2019
		Fenbendazole	Vijayasarathi *et al.*, 2019
Uttar Pradesh	Sheep	Fenbendazole, Tetramisole, Rafoxanide	Singh *et al.*, 2010
	Sheep	Fenbendazole	Kumar *et al.*,2015
	Goat	Fenbendazole, Ivermectin	Kumar *et al.*, 2013
	Equine	Benzimidazole	Kumar *et al.*, 2016
	Goat	Benzimidazole	Chandra *et al.*, 2014
	Sheep	Benzimidazole	Chandra *et al.*, 2015
Uttarakhand	Goat	Fenbendazole	Lahaand Harbola, 1999
	Goat	Albendazole, Rafoxanide	Ram *et al.*, 2007
	Sheep	Fenbendazole, Levamisole, Rafoxanide	Garg *et al.*, 2007
	Sheep	Fenbendazole	Rialch *et al.*, 2013
	Goat	Fenbendazole	
	Goat	Fenbendazole, Tetramisole	Kumar *et al.*, 2017
	Sheep	Fenbendazole, Tetramisole	Kumar *et al.*, 2017

Table 1.2: State-wise Benzimidazole Resistance Report in Livestock in India based on Allele Specific PCR

State	Species	Drug	Reference
Jammu and Kashmir	Goat	Benzimidazole	Bihaqi *et al.*, 2020
Haryana	Sheep	Benzimidazole	Saini *et al.*, 2016
Karnataka	Sheep	Benzimidazole	Adeppa, 2019
Madhya Pradesh	Goat	Benzimidazole	Dixit *et al.*, 2017
Rajasthan	Sheep	Benzimidazole	Tiwari *et al.*, 2006

State	Species	Drug	Reference
Uttar Pradesh	Sheep	Benzimidazole	Chandra *et al.*,2015
	Goat	Benzimidazole	Chandra *et al.*,2014
	Equine	Fenbendazole	Kumar *et al.*, 2016
Uttrakhand	Sheep	Benzimidazole	Garg *et al.*, 2009

Table 1.3: Benzimidazole Resistance in Sheep Based on Restriction Fragment Length Polymorphism PCR

State	Species	Drug	Reference
Rajasthan	Sheep	Benzimidazole	Tiwari *et al.*, 2006, 2006a

Detection of Anthelmintic Resistance

Anthelmintic resistance is detected by number of *in vitro* and *in vivo* detection techniques. Faecal egg count reduction test (FECRT) and egg hatch assay (EHA) are recommended by the World Association for the Advancement of Veterinary Parasitology (WAAVP) as field tests to detect anthelmintic resistance. DrenchRite® Kit larval development assay is the commercially available kit and marketed by Horizon Tech, Australia. It is the most suitable *in vitro* detection method for all broad spectrum anthelmintics (Verma *et al.*, 2018).

In vivo Assays

Faecal Egg Count Reduction Test

At present scenario this test is mostly used and recommended for detecting and monitoring the presence of AR. It is suitable for all types of anthelmintics, against all types of helminths and useful in all host species (Taylor *et al.*, 2002). The basic principle of the test is comparing the egg count of pre-treatment and post-treatment faecal sample. As female worms briefly suppress their egg laying properties the post-treatment faecal egg count should be carried out at 3-4 days, 8-10 days and10-14 days for levamisole, benzimidazoles and avermectins, respectively. FECRT is calculated according to the WAAVP method and the criterion for anthelmintic resistance is FECRT of less than 95 per cent associated with 95 per cent confidence interval extending below the 90 per cent level. Severity of resistance may be classified as moderate when FECRT is between 60-90 per cent and severe with less than 60 per cent FECRT (Coles *et al.*, 2006).

In vitro Assays

Egg Hatch Assay

In this assay, undeveloped eggs are recovered from pooled fresh faecal sample and are incubated in increasing concentration of anthelmintic drugs. The concentration of drug required to inhibit hatching of 50 per cent of nematode eggs is determined by counting all eggs and larvae as dead, embryonated or hatched L1 at each concentration. A dose response line is plotted against the drug concentration. The reference drug used to conduct this test is thiabendazole (Coles *et al.*, 2006).

Larval Development Assay

Larval development assay is used for detecting resistance in benzimidazoles, levamisole and ivermectin resistance. Nematode eggs are isolated from pooled faecal samples and are dispensed into wells of microtitre plate containing a range of anthelmintic drugs. Eggs are allowed to develop into infective L3 and all eggs and larvae are counted. LD50 value (anthelmintic concentration at which 50 per cent larval development is inhibited) is calculated against the number of larvae in the control well and dose response curve is plotted. By comparing the LD50 value of resistant isolates, resistance ratio is determined (Rialch *et al.*, 2013; Verma *et al.*, 2018).

Molecular Assays

Molecular mechanisms of resistance vary for each anthelmintic class. Therefore, different techniques are to be developed for each class of drug. The molecular assays are highly sensitive and less expensive. So far, allele specific PCR, PCR- RFLP, real time PCR are developed for detecting AR in BZs.

Allele Specific PCR

An allele-specific polymerase chain reaction (PCR) was able to detect amino acid substitution (Phe to Tyr) at position 200 in the β-tubulin isotype 1 gene in *H. contortus*, important in conferring benzimidazole resistance. Further, allele-specific PCRs for the genotyping other benzimidazole resistant nematode species in regard to this mutation on position 200 of the β-tubulin gene have been reported (Elard *et al.*, 1999; Silvestre and Humbert, 2000; Chandra *et al.*, 2014, 2015; Dixit *et al.*, 2017). AS-PCR has an advantage over the existing assays in terms of specificity, sensitivity and give quick results with less input.

PCR-Restriction Fragment Length Polymorphisms (RFLPs)

By restriction fragment length polymorphisms (RFLPs), DNA polymorphisms in the genome of benzimidazole susceptible and resistant populations of larval and adult *H. contortus* after Southern blotting was investigated by Roos *et al.*, 1990 in their study. Later, an easy, rapid and sensitive PCR-RFLP technique was described to amplify a PCR product linked RFLP for 200th codon (Tiwari *et al.*, 2006, 2006a) and 167 codon (Shokrani *et al.*, 2012).

Strategies to Delay and Mitigate the Development of Resistance

The problem of AR can be overcome either by delaying its onset or use of alternate strategies in the form of integrated parasite management. The strategies to delay the development of resistance fall under various categories. They are:

Practical Approaches to Minimize AR

Measures such as reduction in drench frequency, rotational use of the drug class, administering appropriate drug doses, use of narrow spectrum of anthelmintics when possible and combined use of drugs from two different classes slow down the selection of resistant worms during early steps of resistance development.

Target selective treatment (TST) is a practical approach based on the refugia concept where the entire animals is not treated, only the selected animals are treated. There are several indicators to selectively target anthelmintic treatment, of which FAMACHA system is the practical and proven method. It is used for the clinical evaluation of anemia in host by comparing the colour of the conjunctival mucosa to a chart. Based on the grade of anaemia, animals those require medical intervention alone are treated. Other indicators are faecal egg counts, dag score, diarrhea score (DISCO), body weight and body condition score (BCS) and performance-based indicators (milk yield, live weight gain). These efforts will slow down further development of resistance but will not reverse the existing resistance in a population.

Nutritional Management

Animals on high protein diet are withstand to parasitic infection. This protein may be obtained from locally available resources, so that cost required for high protein has minimized. Supplementation of cobalt, copper, phosphorus, zinc, iron, molybdenum in the diet boosts the immune system and prevents the establishment of worms (Shalaby, 2013).

Genetic Improvement

Anthelmintic resistance is linked with the inheritance of gene and is moderately heritable 0.2 – 0.4. Use of breeds that are resistant to helmintic infection for cross-breeding would improve the resistance to parasitic infection (Shalaby, 2013). This approach is highly achievable in farm conditions.

Immunological Approaches

Barbervax, first commercially available sub-unit vaccine against barberpole worm, *Haemonchus contortus.* However, multiple doses may be cost effective and not affordable to poor farmers. Other commercially available anti-helmintic vaccines are Difil and Bovilis huskvac.

Bioactive Forages

Plants with higher level of condensed tannins (CT) are referred to as bioactive forages and are said to have anti-parasitic property. Grazing on bioactive forages, such as chicory, oak leaves, guava leaves, jackfruit leaves has been shown to reduce the negative effects of parasitism. These crops must be integrated into the normal diet of ruminants.

Plant-based Anthelmintics

Several reports are available on anthelmintic property of various commonly available plants. Leaf, stem, fruit, root, root barks or extracts of indigenous plants such as *Allium sativum* (Garlic), *Azadirachta indica (Neem)*, *Ferula asafetida (Asafoetida)*, *Zingiber officinale* (Ginger), *Calotropis procera* (giant milkweed), *Piper longum* (Long pepper), *Punica granatum* (Pomegranate), *Carum copticum* (Ajwain), *Agatigratifola* (Agati), *Mangifera indica* (Mango), *Nigella sativa*(Black cumin), *Swertia chirata* (Chiretta), *etc.* have potential anthelmintic property. These plants have been reported to have compounds like saponins, polyphenols, alkaloids, lignins, tannins, catechins, flavonoids, steroids, glycosides and enzymes like cysteine proteases which are responsible for the anthelmintic property (Tariq *et al.*, 2012; Veerakumari, 2015).

There are few commercial herbal dewormers with varied herbal combinations:

- ☆ R- Worm bolus contains *Mallotus philippensis, Embelia ribes, Butea Parviflora, Acacia Arabica, Azadiracta indica, cassia augustifolia, Mesuaferia.*
- ☆ Verm Oust is an all natural herbal wormer feed supplement formulated for horses, cows, goats, sheep, pigs, fowl, and dogs. It contains wormwood, peppermint leaf, gentian root, fennel, psyllium, clove, quassia, olive leaf, turmeric, black walnut, cayenne.
- ☆ Wormikap acts against all common species of gastrointestinal helminths, worms are paralyzed and are expelled in the faeces. It eradicates ova, immature and mature worms, hence reduce the risk of re-infestation, and free from adverse effects.

Chapter 2

In vitro Detection of Anthelmintic Resistance by Egg Hatch Assay (EHA)

S. Nath, R. Verma, S. Kumar and S. Mandal

Department of Veterinary Parasitology,
College of Veterinary Science and Animal Husbandry NDVSU,
Jabalpur – 482001, Madhya Pradesh

Introduction

Anthelmintic resistance is initially suspected when a flock shows poor clinical performance to treatment. Often resistance is not diagnosed properly and continued use of the same anthelmintic group increases the frequency resistance to the level where there is a major failure of control. Resistance is an inevitable phenomenon but regular monitoring and surveillance of benzimidazole resistance status assists in timely implementation of resistance mitigation strategies in farms and field. Egg hatch assay (EHA) evaluates the ability of benzimidazoles to impede or prevent embryonation and hatching of nematode eggs and is the standard *in vitro* test for detection of benzimidazole resistance. Egg Hatch Assay (EHA) was first applied by Le Jambre (1976) as a widespread tool to detect benzimidazole resistance. This was followed by Cawthorne and Cheong (1984), Taylor and Hunt (1988), Swarnkar*et al.* (1999) and several others. The EHA is well validated and provides a more quantitative estimate of benzimidazole resistance. Although it was thiabendazole resistance that was detected by the above workers, Coles *et al.* (1992) have recommended that resistance to other benzimidazole compounds could also be detected by EHA although some benzimidazoles are very insoluble and thus difficult to use. At the same time long-term stability of thiabendazole in solutions of DMSO is not known but reduction in anticipated concentrations may occur when stock solutions are diluted in water. The Egg Hatch Assay describe over here is as per Coles *et al.* (1992; 2006) and it was accepted by World Association for Advancement of veterinary Parasitology (WAAVP). EHA is one of the rapid, economic and convenient detection methods suitable for routine evaluation of benzimidazole resistance both in farm and field animals. The only requirement is trained professional for carrying out the test.

Collection of Faecal Sample

About 5 to 10 gm fresh faecal sample were collected per rectum from each animal in case of small ruminants whereas for horse and other animals freshly laid droppings can be used. Faecal samples may be pooled as per the requirement of the experiment. Sensitivity to thiabendazole decreases with the age of the eggs, therefore, eggs should be used within 3 h of collection. If the laboratory or the testing facility is far away from collection site, eggs can be stored anaerobically (Hunt and Taylor, 1989). For developing anaerobic condition pooled faecal samples should be collected in sample container preferably 100ml to 500ml containing distilled water and about ten 8 mm glass beads. Sample container was screwed tight, almost full with water and shaked vigorously. Store the bottle at room temperature. Do not refrigerate. Eggs for tests can be used up to 7 days after collection. For EHA the part pooled sample collected on the zero day of treatment should be used and not the samples which were collected on the 10th day of treatment when you are doing FECRT simultaneously. Horse samples can be treated similarly but addition of 1 g glucose may increase the onset of anaerobic conditions.

Preparation of Faecal Slurry

The pooled faecal sample maintained in anaerobic condition should be taken in a large size beaker (2 lit) and about 500 ml to 1000 ml water will be added in the beaker. It should be kept for 20-30 minutes so that faecal matter gets soaked and loosened. Faecal material is thoroughly mixed with stirrer. Homogenizing faecal samples until all pellets are broken. After mixing faecal slurry will strained 2-3 times using tea strainer to remove the faecal debris.

Separation of Eggs from Faecal Slurry

Strained faecal slurry is to be poured in centrifuge tubes and centrifuged at 2000 rpm for 5 minutes. After centrifugation supernatant were discarded from all centrifuge tubes. Sediment should be well agitated and saturated sodium chloride solution will be added up to top in each centrifuge tube for floatation of parasitic eggs. Microscopic cover slips will be kept on each centrifuge tube for adhering of eggs. After 10 minutes cover glasses will be lifted with forcep and dipped in a petridish containing distilled water. Take out the cover slip and the egg content will be taken into a conical centrifuge tube. With centrifuges tube where use of a cover slip is difficult the top layer of solution containing egg can be sucked off after centrifugation with a pasteur pipette. Fill the tube with water and centrifuge for 2 min at about 2000 rpm. Remove the water, re-suspend the eggs in water, estimate the numbers of eggs per decimicroliter and dilute to 100–150/100 µl.

Preparation of Thiabendazole Stock Solution

Weigh 10 mg of thiabendazole (TBZ) using precision monopan balance. Thiabendazole should be put in a glass vial. Pour 5ml of di-methyl-sulphoxide (DMSO) to dissolve the drug. This solution will be used as stock solution. By using stock solution five different doses of thiabendazole will be prepared in a two-fold serial dilution by the method as depicted in the Table 2.1.

Table 2.1: Concentration of TBZ in different Tubes with Two-fold Dilution

Tube no.	*1*	*2*	*3*	*4*	*5*
Volume of stock solution (ml)	0.5	-	-	-	-
Volume of D.W. (ml)	4.5	1.0	1.0	1.0	1.0
Volume taken from tube 1 (ml)	-	1.0	-	-	-
Volume taken from tube 2 (ml)	-	-	1.0	-	-
Volume taken from tube 3 (ml)	-	-	-	1.0	-
Volume taken from tube 4 (ml)	-	-	-	-	1.0
Total Volume (ml)	5.0	2.0	2.0	2.0	2.0
Conc.TBZ(µg TBZ/10µl)	2.0	1.0	0.5	0.25	0.125

Charging and Incubation of 24 Multiwell Plate

A twenty fourmultiwell plate is used in this technique. Ten µl of prepared dilutions of TBZ: 0.125, 0.25, 0.5, 1.0 and 2.0 µg/mlwill be added to five different wells in duplicate or can be in triplicate. 10 µl DMSO is added to two wells and kept as control wells. 1.89 ml distilled water (DW) will be added to each well in a 24 multiwell plate. Egg suspension (100 µl) is poured in each well containing TBZ or DMSO. Plates should be covered to prevent drying out and incubate in a BOD incubator at 28°C for 24-48 hr.

Counting of Eggs and Larvae

After 24 hrs of incubation of the multiwell plate, embryonationwill be checked from control wells using 10x objective of compound microscope or stereoscope. If larvae are found in control well, then further processing will be carried out. Solution from different wells are pipetted out and poured in separate centrifuge tubes. Add a drop of Lugol's iodine in each tube to stop further hatching. These tubes are centrifuged at 2000 rpm for 5 min. Supernatant will be discarded very carefully. Aliquot of sediment will be observed for counting of eggs and larvae under 10x objective of compound microscope.Each drug concentration should be tested at least in duplicate.

Interpretation of Data

The mean number of eggs and larvae at each concentration will be calculated and mean per cent hatch inhibition is derived using the following formula.

$$\text{Per cent hatch inhibition} = \frac{\text{Number of eggs}}{\text{No of egg + No of larvae}} \times 100$$

These adjusted percentages were plotted against the drug concentration log10 scale. The EHA data are therefore presented as the mean percentage egg death plotted against the drug concentration on a logarithmic scale. To calculate the 95 per cent confidence intervals, the ED50 values were calculated by using the Probit (probability unit) software which transforms the proportion of egg death to a unit based on the integration of the normal curve distribution to fit a straight line to dosage-mortality data (Busvine, 1971).The data was analysed by Probit Analysis to obtain ED_{50} value for egg hatch by log-probit analysis using SPSS or even with EXCEL programme. A program to calculate the ED_{50} on the egg hatch test is available with many institution such as CSWRI.ED_{50} value in excess of 0.1µg TBZ ml^{-1} will be considered as emergence of TBZ resistance.

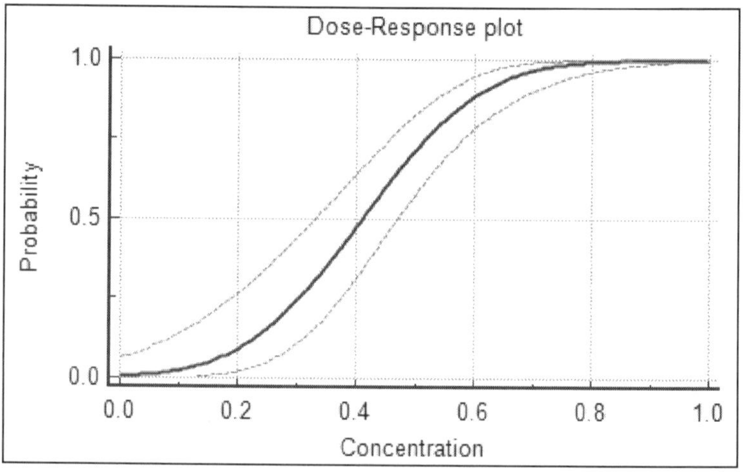

Figure 2.1: Plot of Dose-Response Curve.

Conclusion

Egg hatch assay is most suitable for small ruminants. However, discriminating doses have not been established for eggs from nematodes of cattle and pigs therefore cannot be applied on them. Egg hatch assay is an *in vitro* diagnostic test that can be practiced in surveys for benzimidazole resistance detection in farms and field. The assay is less time taking, less arduous and quicker when compared with other detection tests such as faecal egg count reduction test (FECRT) and larval development assay (LDA). However, conventional tests for resistance detection like EHA have low sensitivity and detect resistance only when the resistant alleles are more than 25 per cent in the population (Taylor *et al.*, 2002). Further, we cannot detect the heterogenic cases of resistance which indeed is one of criteria for making effective strategies for mitigation.

Chapter 3

In vivo Detection of Anthelmintic Resistance

S. Nath, R. Verma, S. Kumar, S. Mandal and G. Das

Department of Veterinary Parasitology,
College of Veterinary Science and Animal Husbandry NDVSU,
Jabalpur – 482001, Madhya Pradesh

Introduction

The detection of anthelmintic resistance (AR) are becoming increasingly important for health programs of grazing livestock (Kaplan and Vidyashankar, 2012). AR is a problem usually associated with conventional production systems,The major *in vivo* method for the detection of resistance remains the faecal egg count reduction test (FECRT) that can be used with all anthelmintic groups. Nematode eggs are counted in faeces at the time of treatment and at defined times after treatment, the time depending on the anthelmintic group used. This test is only reliable if more than 25 per cent of the worms are resistant (Martin *et al.*, 1989). The faecal egg count reduction test (FECRT) was done according to the World Association for the Advancement of Veterinary Parasitology (WAAVP) guidelines for detection of anthelmintic resistance (Coles *et al.*, 1992). However, the methods like Critical evaluation test and Controlled tests are till now gold standards for evaluation of efficacies of different antiparasitic drug groups against different species of parasites for different group of animals.

Faecal Egg Count Reduction Test (FECRT)

Selection of Animals

The maximum number of animals having uniformity in the nature and intensity of nematode infection, age, and weight from each flock were taken in the study. The experimental animals should be naturally parasitized with mixed species of gastrointestinal nematodes {having at least 150 eggs per gram of faeces (EPG)}. It should be ascertained that the selected animals had not been treated in the previous 8-12 weeks. Young animals, 3-6 months of age which have been bred on the property under examination should be given priority. Randomly distribute animals, or distribute by faecal egg counts if practicable, into control and treatment groups of 15 animals each. A control (untreated) group should be used to allow for natural changes in egg counts during the test.

Collection of Faecal Sample

Faecal egg count reduction was the criterion for detection of resistance. About 5 to 10 grams of faecal samples were collected individually directly from rectum into sterile polybags from all animals before treatment and on day 10 of post-treatment. About 3 gms of the collected faecal material was used for FECRT and rest of the samples were pooled as per the place of collection. Faecal examination should be conducted using standard procedures and EPG were counted by a modified McMaster method using McMaster slide. Carry on the process if the group mean egg count is more than 150 EPG. Group mean egg counts below 150 epg can be common in adult sheep. The remaining samples are to be cultured for speciation of nematodes, samples should not be stored at 4 °C as it may affect the hatching of *Haemonchus contortus*.

Treatment

Animals are treated with an anthelmintic according to the manufacturer's recommended dose either as (a) the accurate dose in milligrams per kilogram (for research purposes) or (b) according to the weight of the heaviest animal in the group (for veterinary diagnosis). Dose of benzimidazole is 7.5mg/Kg body weight for suspected closantel resistance in *H. contortus*, 2.5 mg kg- ~ may be used to avoid the action of the drug caused by its persistence in the body (Lyndal-Murphy, 1992). Anthelmintics should be administered with a syringe or a drench gun that has been previously calibrated. Faecal samples should be collected 10-14 days after treatment. A shorter period before sampling may give misleading results with a number of anthelmintics.

Interpretation of Data

Calculate the arithmetic mean, percentage reduction and 95 per cent confidence interval. The arithmetic mean (X) is preferable to the geometric mean as: (a) it is easier to calculate; (b) it provides a better estimate of the worm egg output; (c) it is a more conservative measure of anthelmintic efficacy. The percentage reduction is 100 (1 -Xt/Xc) where t is the treated group egg count at 10-14 days and c is the control group at 10-14 days. A computer programme, RESO, is available for this calculation.

The faecal egg count data was analysed for faecal egg count reduction (per cent FECR) using RESO calculator (Martin and Wursthorn, 1991) and resistance to anthelmintic is considered if (a) the FECR is <95 per cent and (b) the lower 95 per cent confidence interval is less than 90 per cent. If only one of the two criteria is met resistance is suspected (Coles *et al.*, 1992).

Diagnosis of Genus of the Nematode Present

The genus and species of the nematodes that are resistant to the anthelmintics should be determined. Third-stage larvae are therefore cultured from the eggs in faeces from controls and from treated groups separately.

Coproculture

About 75-100 gm of group-wise pooled faecal material is grounded, mixed with little amount of water to hold sufficient moisture and coprocultured by petri-plate method. The faecal mixture is placed in an incubator set at 25-28°C for 6 days for development of infective third stage larvae. This coproculture is done in both zero day and 10to 14 day of the post-treatment.

Recovery of Larvae

After 6-10 days of culture, the water in the petridish should be pipetted out in a centrifuge tube, labeled individually and centrifuged at 1000 rpm for 2 minutes. The supernatant will be removed and the sediment will beheated by passing through flame of spirit lamp to kill the larvae. Preserve the larvae in 10 per cent formalin. A drop of preserved larval material is placed on a glass slide and mixed with a drop of Lugol's Iodine and examined under microscope for larval micrometry (Skernman and Hillard, 1966).

Larval Identification

Identification of larvae will done as per the keys given in table (Skernman and Hillard, 1966).

1	No sheath, oesophagus half the length of the body	*Strongyloides* spp.
	Sheathed larvae, oesophagus short	2
2	Total length <600μ	*Bunostomum* spp.
	Total length >600μ	3
3	Length of tail sheath <40μ	*Trichostrongylus* spp
	Length of tail sheath >40μ	4
4	Length of tail sheath >140μ	*Oesophagostomum* spp.
	Length of tail sheath >40μ and <140μ	5

5	One or two chitinized inverted "**U**" shaped structures at the anterior end of oesophagus	*Mecistocirrus* spp.
	No inverted "**U**" shaped structures at the anterior end of oesophagus	6
6	Chitinous knobs or spots at the anterior end of oesophagus	*Cooperia* spp.
7	No such structures at the anterior end of oesophagus	*Haemonchus* spp.

Cattle

Groups of 10 animals should be used. These need not be calves providing egg counts are above 150 epg. There are only two reports of resistant nematodes isolated from cattle in the field that have been confirmed by dose and slaughter trials (Eagleson and Bowie, 1986; Jackson *et al.*, 1987). Until further strains of resistant nematodes have been isolated from cattle it is unwise to conclude that a failure to produce a less than 90 per cent reduction in egg count is associated with anthelmintic resistance.

Horses

Animals will often be in very small groups and control groups may not be practical. Resistance in horses is primarily confined to benzimidazoles and is most commonly reported in cyathostomes (small strongyles). A reduction in egg count of less than 90 per cent is indicative of benzimidazole resistance (Bauer *et al.*, 1986).

Pigs

Groups of 10 animals should be used. The only resistance reported is to levamisole/pyrantel in *Oesophagostomum* sp. (Roepstorff*et al.*, 1987; Bjorn *et al.*, 1990). Sows carry the heaviest infection and should be used in tests for anthelmintic resistance with this genus of nematode. A reduction in egg count of less than 90 per cent is indicative of anthelmintic resistance.

Controlled Efficacy and Critical Tests

Both the controlled and critical tests have been widely used and are acceptable in assessing the efficacy and resistance of anthelmintics against many important parasitic helminths of horses, ruminants and other monogastric animals. In most cases, naturally infected animals may be used but it may be desirable in some cases to study drug activity against a number of important species, such as some of the large strongyles, by experimental infections.

Controlled Efficacy Test (CET)

In this test, the efficacy of an anthelmintic is determined by comparing parasite populations in groups of treated and untreated animals. This test is the most reliable method for evaluating anthelmintic activity in ruminants and is recommended for dose titration and dose confirmation trials. Parasitized animals are randomly separated into medicated and non-medicated (control) groups and at a suitable interval after treatment are necropsied and the parasites are recovered identified and counted. The use of a placebo control is not required. The following formula expresses the percent efficacy (per cent E) of a dose against a given parasite species (S) in a single treatment group (T) when compared with an untreated control

$$\text{Per cent E} = \frac{\text{Mean of S in C- Mean of S in T}}{\text{Mean of S in C}} \times 100$$

Or worm count reduction percentage (WCR per cent) = 100 × (1 – [T/C]) where

T" is the geometric mean worm count of treatment groups and "C" the geometric mean worm count of the control group.

The geometric mean should be used as it more accurately represents the distribution of nematode populations within a group of animals and would give a more accurate indication of the degree of efficacy of a product.

In the CET total worm counts of each nematode species were log-transformed for comparison between groups using a one-way ANOVA with a Bonferroni post hoc test. Efficacy of a given anthelmintic treatment to remove adult nematodes from the animals was calculated as worm count reduction percentage (WCR per cent) = 100 × (1 – [T/C]) (Wood *et al.*, 1995; Bartley *et al.*, 2004). Using the method of Wood *et al.* (1995), "T" is the geometric mean worm count of treatment groups and "C" the geometric mean worm count of the control group. According to Wood *et al.* (1995), an anthelmintic is highly effective if the WCR per cent is >98 per cent, effective when the WCR per cent is 90–98 per cent, moderately effective if WCR per cent is 80–89 per cent and insufficiently effective if the WCR per cent is <95 per cent.

Critical Tests

In this test, efficacy is determined by comparing the numbers of parasites eliminated in the feces from an animal after treatment with the number remaining in the animal at necropsy. This method is often used for trials with monogastric animals such as dogs, horses and swine where the parasites generally are eliminated in identifiable condition (Duncan *et al.*, 2002). The critical test is not recommended for evaluation of anthelmintics against most nematodes in ruminants, but may be considered for trials with large bowel parasites *e.g. Oesophagostomum* and *Chabertia* which may be eliminated intact in the faeces.

Although time-consuming and laborious this method may be used to assess efficacy against lumen dwelling gastrointestinal parasites using individual infected animals which act as their own controls. The animals are maintained singly and dosed with a test compound. Faeces are collected daily from 1 day before to up to at least 7 days after administration of the drug when the animal is killed and necropsied. The parasites are collected from the daily faecal output and at necropsy those remaining in the gastrointestinal tract are recovered, identified and counted. The total of these collections is considered to be the worm burden which existed at the time of treatment, and the efficacy against any particular species in each individual animal is calculated from the following data

$$\text{Percent efficacy} = \frac{\text{Number of Parasite expelled}}{\text{No. of Parasite expelled + No. of Parasite remaining at necropsy}} \times 100$$

A disadvantage of this test is that small nematodes normally found in the stomach or small intestine may be partially digested when passed in the faeces and thus are difficult to find or identify. The use of the critical test for efficacy data against such parasites will therefore result in a conservative estimate of efficacy. Accuracy will also be affected by natural losses of parasites during the faecal collection period. The pooled results from several critical tests may give sufficient data for registration of a compound against individual parasite species. Both controlled and critical tests may be used to assess efficacy against adult, and larval stages where appropriate, for example in the case of larval stages present in the lumen of the gastrointestinal tract. The controlled test, using natural or experimental infections, is suitable for determining efficacy against larval stages which are not in the lumen of the intestine. In this case, necropsy may be delayed to allow immature parasites in the controls and those which have survived treatment, to mature and thus facilitate collection and identification.

Artificially Induced Infections

These are preferred for dose titration trials and can be used in dose confirmation trials. Induced infections may be superimposed upon natural infections to ensure adequate numbers of the more important species and for concurrent testing against a wide range of nematodes. Induced infections are generally necessary to determine and confirm efficacy against immature stages of parasites and adults of less common species. These infections should be established in young, nematode-naive calves, lambs or kids in good health. Suckling animals should not be used. Before infection, animals should be examined for internal parasites and, if infected, treated with double the therapeutic dose of a broad spectrum non-persistent anthelmintic chemically unrelated to the one being tested. After treatment, feces should be examined to ensure the animals are helminth-free and the animals held for 1-2 weeks prior to infection. Generally, avermectins, milbemycins or related agents should not be used because of their persistent activity. If these are necessary, at least 1 month must elapse after treatment before the induced infection. Animals with induced infections should be confined under drylot or other conditions which preclude further exposure to infective larvae. The reasons for the decision to select induced infections, the source, characteristics, number of laboratory passages and method of storage or maintenance of infective larvae (L 3) should be documented.

Conclusion

Among the three *in vivo* tests for detection of anthelmintic resistance the most prevalent is FECRT due to its simplicity and effective implication. Moreover this method is also applied due to its ethical approval

Chapter 4

Molecular Detection of Anthelmintic Resistance

M. Sankar, K.A.Yashica, V.K, Tiwari, V. Prasanth, M. Silamparasan, R. Garg and S. Ghosh

Indian Veterinary Research Institute, Izatnagar – 243122, Uttar Pradesh

Aim and Target

Early diagnosis of benzimidazole resistance in strongylesby allele specific PCR (AS-PCR).

Principle

AS-PCR is one of the competitive PCRs, mainlyused for diagnosing single nucleotide polymorphism (SNP)/point mutation. It is also called as arm PCR. The amplification is based on the variations of the primers at the 3′ end, which has been designed such a way that to amplify for wild/mutant, accordingly. Thus, the modifications of the primers on 3′ end amplifyamplify the normal allele and the mutant allele. This mismatch on 3′ end of a primer allows to anneal one single allele. AS-PCR generally contains more than three primers, two internal control primers (forward and reverse non allele specific) and any one of allele specific (wild/mutant) in case of three primer strategy and two internal control primers (forward and reverse non allele specific) and two allele specific primers (both wild and mutant) in case of four primer strategy. However, four primers strategy has limitations of cross-annealing in most related species of a genus.

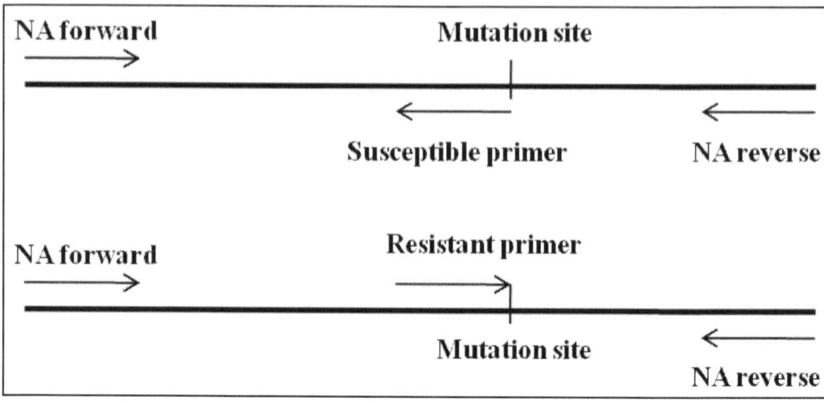

Schematic Diagram of AS-PCR Strategy.

Materials Required for Performing AS-PCR

Equipment/Glass Wares/Plastic Wares

- ☆ Binocular microscope
- ☆ Dissection microscope
- ☆ Autoclave/cooker
- ☆ 4 °C refrigerator
- ☆ -20 °C refrigerator
- ☆ Thermal cycler
- ☆ Electrophoresis unit and power pack
- ☆ Gel documentation
- ☆ Hot water Bath
- ☆ Centrifuge
- ☆ Weighing balance
- ☆ Micropipettes of various volumes
- ☆ Vortexer
- ☆ Microtips of 10 µl, 200 µl, 1000 µl
- ☆ Eppendorf tubes of 1.5 ml, 2.0 ml
- ☆ PCR tubes of 0.2 ml
- ☆ Petridishes
- ☆ Pipet stand
- ☆ Boxes for Eppendorf and PCR tubes
- ☆ Cryopreservation tubes and boxes

Chemicals/Reagents Required

- Phosphate buffered saline (pH 7.4)
- Sodium hypochrolite(3.5-4 per cent active chlorine)
- Ethanol
- Tris Base
- Ethylene diamine tetra acetic acid (EDTA)
- Proteinase K
- Nonidet-P 40
- Taq DNA polymerase
- Deoxyribonucleotide triphosphate (dNTP)
- Oligonucleotides primers
- DNA markers
- Glacial acetic acid
- Boric acid
- 6x gel loading dye
- Nuclease free water
- Agarose
- Ethidium bromide
- Restriction enzyme *RsaI*
- Cotton (absorbable)/tissue paper

Biological Materials

Adult Parasites

Collect adult parasites from GI tract of sheep and goat slaughtered at local abattoir/meat shop. Wash the parasites thoroughly in PBS (PH 7.4) and identify as per the morphological keys. Use adult parasite for DNA isolation or preserved in 70 per cent ethanol and store at -20°C for further use.

Larvae

Prepare faeces culture by adding three parts of sterilized powdered faeces and two parts of activated charcoal powder or simple sterilized/autoclaved powdered faeces. Put the mixture over an inverted positioned small petridish. Keep small petridish in a large petridish containing distilled water. Cover the large petridish by another petridish of same size to avoid entrance of fly/dirt particles and other contaminants. Implant the sample eggs/triturated adult female worm on the surface of the culture. Incubate the culture at room temperature (28-35 °C) and check the larvae in the culture regularly. Normally, the infective larvae appear within 4-6 days. The protozoan contamination avoids by changing the distilled water once a day up to 5th day of culture.

Genomic DNA Extraction from Adult/Single Larvae

The protocol for isolation of genomic DNA described in Coles *et al.* (2006) with minor modifications. Wash larvae 3-4 times with distilled water, and exshealth in sodium hypochlorite (4 per cent active chlorine) for 20- 30 min (35 µl of sodium hypochlorite/ml of water VV per cent). Collect single exshealthed larva (under microscope) by micropipette and kill by placing in a micro tube at –20°C for 20 min. Extract DNA by adding 5µl digestion buffer (100 mM Tris-HCl, 10 mM EDTA and 5mg/ml proteinase K or Nonidet P 40 buffer from Amresco) and incubate tubes at 56°C for 4-6 hrs. Use 20 µl of digestion buffer for adult parasites. Inactivate proteinase K by incubate at 95°C for 20 minutes. This step is more crucial as presence of proteinase K interfere downstream function. Centrifuge (in refrigerated centrifuge is preferable) the lysate at 4000 rpm for 2 min and use 5 µl of supernatant for fragment of β-tubulin isotype-1 gene (target gene for BZ resistance).

Amplification of Fragment of β-tubulin Iso Type 1 Gene

Perform PCR in 25 µl reaction volume. The PCR mixture consist of 10-20pmoles of each primer (Pn_1 and Pn_2) (Table 4.1), 1mM $MgCl_2$, 100µM of each dNTPs, and 1U of Taq DNA polymerase with 10x Taq DNA polymerase buffer. Perform reaction with annealing temperature at 57°C. To reduce the cost of the assay, the reaction volume may be reduced with 12.5 µl.

Table 4.1: Primers Details for Primary, Nested and AS-PCR

PCR	*Primers*	*Annealing Temperature*
Primary PCR	Pn1 GGC AAA TAT GTC CCA CGT GC	57 °C
	Pn2 GAA GCG CGA TAC GCT TGA GC	20 cycles
Nested PCR	Pn3 GTG CTG TTC TTG TTG ATC TC	55 °C/57 °C
	Pn3 GTG CTG TTC TTG TTG ATC TC	33 cycles
AS-PCR for *H. contortus*	Ph1 forward primer GGA ACG ATG GAC TCC TTT CG	55 °C
	Ph2 reverse primer GGG AAT CGA AGG CAG GTC GT	33 cycles
	Ph3 resistant primer CTG GTA GAG AAC ACC GAT GAA ACA TA	
	Ph4 susceptible primer ATA CAG AGC TTC GTT GTC AAT ACA GA	

Nested PCR

Use theprimary PCR amplicons as template for nested PCR. The PCR mixture consist of 1.0 µl of β-tubulin amplicons (primary PCR),15-20pmoles of Pn_3 and Pn_4 primers, 100 µM of each dNTPs, 2mM of $MgCl_2$, 2.5µl of 10x Taq DNA polymerase buffer and 1 U of Taq DNA polymerase.

RFLP with *RsaI* Enzyme

Digest 10 µl of nested amplicons with the restriction enzyme *RsaI* for species identification in case of larva. Perform restriction enzyme digestion for 4 hours in water at 37°C (normal enzyme)/30 min to 1 hr (fast digest enzyme). Resolve the digested fragments by electrophoresis on a 2.5 per cent agarose gel and their digested amplicon lengths used for species identification. Restriction digests yield *H. contortus* of 440, 190 and 140 bp, and *T. colubriformis* yield four major fragments of 390, 180, 100 and 40 bp.

Allele Specific PCR

The current protocol is following three primer strategy. Use two aliquots (1.0 µl) of the nested product to determine the resistance of larvae/adult against BZ group of drugs. The reactions divide into two mixes, each containing two non-allele specific primers and one of allele specific primers. Each reaction generates one allele specific and one non - allele specific fragments. The PCR mixture volume is 25µl, which consists of 7.5pmoles of Ph1/Pc1 and Ph2/Pc2 (non allele specific primers), 25pmoles of Ph3/Pc3in one mix and Ph4/Pc4in another mix, 2mM $MgCl_2$, 80µM of each dNTPs, 2.5µl of Taq DNA polymerase buffer and 1U of Taq DNA polymerase. The resulting fragments is to be separated by gel electrophoresis in a 2.5 per cent agarose gel in TAE (1x) buffer for 1 hour at constant voltage (100V). The non allele specific amplicons yield 750 bp and resistant alleles yield 222 and 250 bp for *H. contortus* and *T. colubriformis*, respectively. The susceptible allele yields 602 bp for *H. contortus* and 550 bp for *T. colubriformis*. Based on AS-PCR, estimate the allele frequency of homozygous susceptible/resistant and heterozygous susceptible based on residue 200 (Phe or Tyr) of isotype 1 b-tubulin gene.

REFERENCES

Chandra, S., Prasad, A., Yadav, N., Latchumikanthan, A., Rakesh, R.L., Praveen, K., Khobra, V., Subramani, K.V., Misri, J. and Sankar, M., 2015. Status of benzimidazole resistance in Haemonchus contortus of goats from different geographic regions of Uttar Pradesh, India. Veterinary Parasitology, 208(3-4), pp.263-267.

Coles, G. C., Jackson, F., Pomroy, W. E., Prichard, R. K., Samson-Himmelstjerna, G. V., Silvestre, A., Taylor M. A. and Vercruysse, J. (2006). The detection of anthelmintic resistance in nematodes of veterinary importance. *Veterinary Parasitology*, 136: 167-185.

Dixit, A.K., Das, G., Dixit, P., Singh, A.P., Kumbhakar, N.K., Sankar, M. and Sharma, R.L., 2017. An assessment of benzimidazole resistance against caprine nematodes in Central India. Tropical animal health and production, 49(7), pp.1471-1478.

Silvestre, A. and Humbert, J.F. (2000). A molecular tool for species identification and benzimidazole resistance diagnosis in larval communities of small ruminant parasites. *Experimantal Parasitol*ogy, 95: 271-276.

Chapter 5

Anthelmintic Resistance and its Mitigation Strategies

G. Das, S. Kumar, S. Nath, R. Verma, R.K. Khare and V. Punia

College of Veterinary Science and Animal Husbandry, NDVSU, Jabalpur – 482001, Madhya Pradesh

Introduction

Livestock can be infected with a variety of helminths on pastures, through ingestion of the larvae of the parasites on the contaminated grass, the most common of which are gastrointestinal nematodes. Helminths have constantly been problematic and a long-standing concern that threatens the livestock industry throughout the world and these parasites has a negative impact on animal productivity, feed intake, growth rate and milk yield. The intensive use of anthelmintics for control of GI nematodes has resulted in the widespread development of resistance to one or more of the widely used anthelmintics in many countries. With few new drugs or vaccine, the fight against parasites could become a losing battle. Understanding the development of drug resistance in parasitic helminths is crucial to prolong the efficacy of current anthelmintics and developing markers for monitoring drug resistance. It has been observed that frequent usage of the same group of anthelmintic; use of anthelmintics in sub-optimal doses, prophylactic mass treatment of domestic animals and frequent and continuous use of a single drug have contributed to the widespread development of anthelmintic resistance in helminths. Today anthelmintic resistance is recognized as a problem worldwide involving the main anthelmintic families. Despite notable activity to develop new anthelmintic classes but the chances of release of a product with a new mode of action in near future is gloomy. Even, new drugs are developes. Resistance will also be developed in due course.

Therefore, it is of utmost importance to find better ways to use the anthelmintic substances we are having in judicial manner preserving their efficacy as long as possible.

What is Anthelmintic Resistance (AR)?

For decades anthelmintics have been used as the primary control measure for worm infecting livestock. However, there has been continuous development of anthelmintic resistance (AR) by the parasitic worms. The definition of resistance varies in different publications. Anthelmintic resistance can be defined as the ability of parasites to survive doses of drugs that would normally kill parasites of the same species and stage. It is inherited and selected for because the survivors of treatments pass genes for resistance onto their offspring. These resistant genes are initially rare in the population or arise as rare mutations, but as selection continues, their proportion in the population increases as does the proportion of resistant parasites. Resistance is the heritable (and therefore genetic) ability of the worm to survive treatment with an anthelmintic. A worm is said to be resistant if it survives exposure to the standard recommended dose of the anthelmintic. Anthelmintic resistance is said to exist in a population of worms if more than 5 per cent of the worms survive treatment. However, unless you test for resistance you will not notice the increasing lack of effectiveness of treatment until 50 per cent or more of the worms survive, at which point the production losses are significant. However, as stated by Coles, resistance occurs when a susceptible population shows any decrease in response to treatment and is complete when the maximum dose that can be tolerated by the host has no effect.

The following definition is given by the World Association for the Advancement of Veterinary Parasitology (WAAVP) is a failure to reduce faecal nematode egg count by at least 95 per cent. Technically accurate definition is that resistance is a genetically determine decline in the efficacy of an anthelmintic against a population of parasite that is susceptible to the drug.

Prevalence of Anthelmintic Resistance

The history of parasite resistance to anthelmintics starts with the first report on phenothiazine resistance in 1957. *H. contortus* was the first nematode to develop resistance against the different anthelmintics. Benzimidazoles are the oldest class of authorized anthelmintics; thiabendazole was introduced in the 1960s. The first report of decreased efficacy of thiabendazole against *H. contortus* strains dates from 1964, just 3 years after its introduction to the market (Table 5.1).

Table 5.1: Introduction of Anthelmintic Drugs for Ruminants and the Development of Resistance to the Drug

Anthelmintic	*Mode of action*	*Mechanism of resistance*	*Generic Drug Name*	*Introduced on the Market*	*Resistance Reported*
Benzimidazole	Inhibiting polymerization of microtubules	Altered target structure (β-tubulin isotype 1 mutations)	Thiabendazole	1961	1964 (USA, 1964 *H. contortus*)
		β -tubulin isotype 2 mutations, deletion, Altered metabolism and/ or uptake	Albendazole	1972	1983
Imidazothiazoles	Agonist of nicotinergic	Changes in nicotinic acetylcholine receptors-	Levamisole	1970	1979 (Australia, 1976 *H. contortus*)
Tetrahydopyrimidines	Acetylcholine receptors	-	Pyrantel	1974	1996
Macrocyclic lactones	Allosteric modulators of the glutamate-gated chloride channels	Mutations in GluCl and/or GABA-R genes Overexpression of P-glycoproteins Altered target (structure of Glu Cl channel and subunits)	Ivermectin	1981	1988 (S. Africa, 1987 *H. contortus*)
Amino- acetonitrile derivative	Allosteric modulator of AchR (MPTL-1), agonist	-	Monepantel	2009	2013 (New Zealand, *Teladorsagia circumcincta* and *Trichostrongylus colubriformis*)
Spiroindol	Interfere, b-subtype, nAchR, antagonist	-	Derquantel	2010	2011 (New Zealand, *H. contortus*)

The problem of anthelmintic resistance in GI nematode of Ruminant is worldwide and well documented reports of anthelmintic resistance have been made from South Africa, Australia, New Zealand, Malaysia, Spain, France, Denmark, UK, Brazil, and the United States. In India, the first report of anthelmintic resistance in *H. contortus* to phenothiazine and thiabendazole in sheep from State Sheep and Wool Research Station, Pashulok, Rishikesh, U.P. (now in Uttarakhand) was by Varshney and Singh. The prevalence of anthelmintic resistance in India is presented in Table 5.2.

Table 5.2: Prevalence of Anthelmintic Resistance in India

Anthelmintic	*Generic Drug Name*	*Host*	*Species*	*Place*
Benzimidazole		Sheep	Strongyles	Karnataka
		Goat	*H. contortus*	Uttar Pradesh
		Horse	Equine Cyathostomins	Uttar Pradesh
		Goat	Strongyles	Kerala
		Goat	Strongyles	Madhya Pradesh
		Sheep	*H. contortus* and *Teladorsagia* spp.	Tamil Nadu
	Albendazole (ALB)	Sheep	*H. contortus*	Rajasthan
		Sheep	*H. contortus*	Tamil Nadu
		Goat	Strongyles	Gujarat
		Goat	Strongyles	Chhattisgarh
	Fenbendazole	Sheep	*H. contortus*	Haryana
		Goat	*H. contortus*	Haryana
		Sheep	*H. contortus*	Haryana
		Sheep	*H. contortus*	Tamil Nadu
		Goat	Strongyles	Madhya Pradesh
	Mebendazole	Goat	*H. contortus*	Haryana
Tetrahydopyri-midines	Closantel	Sheep	*H. contortus*	Tamil Nadu
	Morantel	Goat	*H. contortus*	Haryana
		Sheep	*H. contortus*	Haryana
Imidazo-thiazoles	levamisole (LEV)	Goat	*H. contortus*	Haryana
		Sheep	*H. contortus* and *Teladorsagia* spp.	Tamil Nadu
		Sheep	*H. contortus*	Haryana
		Goat	Strongyles	Madhya Pradesh
		Goat	Strongyles	Gujarat
		Goat and Cattle	Strongyles	Chhattisgarh

Anthelmintic	Generic Drug Name	Host	Species	Place
Macrocyclic lactones	Ivermectin (IVM)	Goat	Strongyle	Gujarat
		Goat and Cattle	Strongyles	Chhattisgarh
		Sheep	*H. contortus*	Haryana

Mechanism of Development of Anthelmintic Resistance

The development of anthelmintic resistance is a complex theme and many factors are involved in the process of resistance selection. In general, anthelmintics are used at an efficacy of around 99.9 per cent against susceptible strains. The few numbers of surviving worms, which are the most resistant component of the population, then infect the pasture with resistant offspring for next generations. There are following three intrinsic phases in the selection process which are linked to the accumulation of resistant alleles:

- **Susceptibility phase:** When the frequency of resistant individuals within the population is low and occurs when the anthelmintic was used initially.
- **Intermediate phase:** It develops following continued exposure to a drug where the frequency of heterozygous resistant individuals within the population increases.
- **Resistant phase:** It is an outcome of sustained selection pressure where homozygous resistant individuals predominate within the population. The speed of this process will depend on how severe the selection pressure is on the parasite population. Under-dosing, which is a common problem, is likely to favour the survival of heterozygous individuals, possibly enhancing the selection pressure for resistance.

Factors Contributing to Development of Anthelmintic Resistance

The rate of development of anthelmintic resistance is influenced by biological, environmental and managemental factor.

Biological Factor

Parasites have short generation time and a well high prolificacy. So there is high increase in generation with spread of resistance alleles in the population. Therefore, their life cycle contributes resistance. Frequent treatments are instituted to control highly pathogenic worms subjecting them to higher selection pressure resulting in quick emergence of anthelmintic resistance. Contrary to that, hypobiotic worms escape the exposure of drug and contribute greatly to refugia population.

Environmental Factors

Climatic conditions determine the type of parasites prevalent and propagate in a particular area. Heavy worm burden during wet season may require higher anthelmintic intervention and this can select rapidly for resistance.

Managemental Factors

Managemental factors are found responsible for emergence of anthelmintic resistance at higher rate.

1. **Drench Frequency:** It has been observed that frequent usage of the same group of anthelmintic may result in the development of anthelmintic resistance.
2. **Under dosing:** Under dosing is generally considered an important factor in the development of anthelmintic resistance because sub therapeutic doses might allow the survival of heterozygous resistant worms.
3. **Continuous use of drug with similar mode of action:** Frequent and continuous use of a single drug leads to the development of resistance. For example, a single drug, which is usually very effective in the first years, is continuously used until it no longer works.
4. **Targeting and timing of mass treatment:** Prophylactic mass treatments of domestic animals have contributed to the widespread development of anthelmintic resistance in helminths. Computer models indicate that the development of resistance is delayed when 20 per cent of the flock is left untreated but it needs confirmation through experimentation.

Detection Methods of Anthelmintic Resistance

Resistance cannot be measured on the basis of an apparent clinical failure to anthelmintic treatment. Other reasons could make clinical signs similar to those normally associated with nematode diseases. Therefore, detection methods are an important means to prove if resistance to an anthelmintic compound is true. Different *in vivo* and *in vitro* tests are now available and there is an ongoing effort to refine, standardize and validate these tests.

Bioassays for the Detection of Anthelmintic Resistances

	Detection of Resistance to	*Application*
A. IN VIVO Tests		
FECRT (Faecal Egg Count Reduction Test)	All	Widespread
Controlled Slaughter Test	Anthelmintic	Limited

	Detection of Resistance to	Application
B. *IN VITRO* Tests		
Egg Hatch Assay	BZ/LEV/MT	
Larval Paralysis Assay	Levamisole/Morantel	Widespread
Tubulin Binding Assay	Benzimidazoles	Limited
Larval Development Assay	All drugs	Commercialized
Adult Development Assay	Benzimidazoles	Limited
Molecular Based Test	All drugs	Limited

1. **Faecal egg count reduction test (FECRT):** This is the most common test to study anthelmintic resistance. The ability of the anthelmintic in question to reduce the concentration of eggs per gram of faeces (EPG) by more than 95 percent, measured 10-14 days after treatment, in comparison with the EPG measured at the time of treatment. Failure to do so is indicative of resistance. This test was originally designed for sheep, but can be used also for cattle, swine and horses. Cut-off value for drug efficacy in FECRT 95 per cent and 90 per cent, macrolides and benzimidazoles/pyrantel, respectively.
2. **Controlled slaughter test:** In this test, the efficacy of an anthelmintic is determined by comparing parasite populations in groups of treated and non-treated animals. Basically, the procedure compares worm burdens of animals artificially infected with susceptible or suspected resistant isolates of nematodes.
3. **Egg hatch assay:** It is based on the determination of the proportion of eggs that fail to hatch in solutions of increasing drug concentration in relation to the control wells, enabling the user of the test to develop a dose response line plotted against the drug concentration. The reference drug used to conduct this test is thiabendazole.
4. **Larval paralysis:** This assay discriminates between resistant and susceptible strains of parasites, by estimating the proportion of third stage larvae in tonic paralysis after incubation with a range of levamisole and morantel drug concentrations.
5. **Tubulin binding assay:** The test is based on the differential binding of benzimidazoles to tubulin, an intracellular structural protein from susceptible and resistant nematodes. Tubulin binding assay involves the incubation of a crude tubulin extract from adult parasites, infective larvae or eggs, with a titrated benzimidazole until equilibrium is reached.
6. **Larval development assay (LDA):** Nematode eggs are isolated from a faecal sample, placed into wells of a microtitre plate and allowed to develop through to infective L_3 larvae in the presence of a range of

concentrations of anthelmintic. The LDA is detection of resistance to benzimidazoles, levamisoles and macrocyclic lactones in nematodes parasites of sheep, horses, pigs and cattle.

DrenchRite® Kit Larvae development assay developed and marketed as DrenchRite® kit (Horizon Tech, Australia) claimed as most suitable *in vitro* detect anthelmintic resistance among all major broad spectrum anthelmintics.

7. **Adult development assay:** The adult development assay for detecting benzimidazole resistance in trichostrongylid nematodes has advanced significantly and *H. contortus* has been cultured through to the adult egg-laying stages, although this test is mainly for research purposes.
8. **Molecular based tests:** The most common molecular mechanism that confers benzimidazole resistance in trichostrongyles in small ruminants involves a phenylalanine to tyrosine mutation at residue 200 of the isotype 1 β-tubulin gene. However, in addition a similar mutation at codon 167 may be involved in benzimidazole resistance in nematodes. An allele-specific polymerase chain reaction (AS-PCR) has been used to detect this mutation in *H. Contortus* and *Teladorsagia circumcincta* adult and larval stage.

Management Strategies to Delay the Development of Resistance

The key areas of concern in the management of anthelmintic resistant throughout the world are: a. Drug related factors (pharmacokinetics, formulation and mode of application of anthelmintics). **b.** Management related factors (incorrect dosing of anthelmintics, frequency of anthelmintic treatment, and use of the same anthelmintic class for several years, pasture management of livestock). **c.** Parasite related factors (number of nematodes in refugia, frequency of genes for resistance in an unselected parasite population, genetic factors as mode of inheritance, fitness and fecundity of resistant nematodes, generation time).

Treatment Strategies

1. **Correct use of anthelmintics:** Under dosing and/or too frequent use of anthelmintics belonging to the same class will increase the risk for selection of resistance.
2. **Reduction in frequency of treatment:** Selection occurs at faster rate with increasing frequency of treatment due to high selection pressure.
3. **Rotational use of anthelmintic:** From the experiment on the frequent use of the same anthelmintics, it has been demonstrated that the alteration of the anthelmintic family may slow down the selection of benzimidazole resistant worms during early steps of resistance development.

4. **A combination drug strategy:** Treating simultaneously with 2 drugs from different anthelmintic classes is one method of preventing the development of anthelmintic resistance.
5. **Using optimum dose:** Under dosing occurs when a host is administered a weight-dependent dose that is less than recommended by the manufacturer and it results from misestimating of body weight. Proper check must be done for calibration of drenching device.
6. **Regular monitoring of anthelmintic resistance:** Regular annual testing with *in vivo* or *in vitro* test is required on farm to monitor the status of drug efficacy of anthelmintics.
7. **Targeted selective treatment (TST):** Targeted selective treatment can be defined as any system that selects animals on an individual basis for treatment, using logical specific criteria on which this selection is made. One in which only those animals that will most benefit from treatment are given anthelmintic. For TST to be viable there must be practical tools that producers can use to make deworming decisions the first tool developed was the FAMACHA system, the Five Point Check is an extension of the FAMACHA system. In the TST group, only 20 per cent of the flock required treatment at any one time and moreover 88 per cent of the animals that were given anthelmintic showed a positive response in performance following treatment:

Check Point	*Observation*	*Possibilities*
1. Eye	Anaemia, 1-5 (FAMACHA© card) (3-5)	*Haemonchus,* Liver fluke, Hook worms and other diseases
2. Back	Condition score 1–5 (BCS card) (1-2)	*Teladorsagia, Trichostrongylus Oesophagostomum,* and other worms
3. Tail	Faecal soiling 1-5 (Dag score card) (3-5)	*Teladorsagia, Trichostrongylus Oesophagostomum,* Flukes and other worms
4. Jaw	Soft swelling	*Haemonchus,* liver fluke Hook worms and other diseases
5. Nose	Discharge	*Oestrus ovis,* Lungworms and other

Alternative Anthelmintic Treatments

Copper-Oxide Wire Particles

Non-chemical strategies to control internal parasites in animals, with these introduced non-chemical approaches form the framework for the livestock health and welfare regarding parasites. The basic principal of this treatment is that the availability of macro-minerals and trace elements influences the host-parasite relationship. When copper-oxide wire particles (COWP) are administered they remain in the rumen and release free copper into the abomasum this free copper particle creates an environment that affects the establishment of *H. contortus* in the abomasum. Copper oxide is available for cattle as a supplement to copper deficiency and has been used in sheep for the same purpose. Optimal dosage is 0.5-2 gm as a single dose to be sufficient to result in reduced FEC. Other chemicals which are having similar activity are diatomaceous earth (DE), copper sulphate and nicotine sulphate.

2. Use of Herbal Anthelmintic

Plants or plant parts with anthelmintic activity are used in folk veterinary medicine, but it is necessary to investigate and scientifically validate low-cost phytotherapeutic alternatives for future use to control GI nematodes in animal by farmers. Indigenous plants like *Areca catechu, Artemisia vulgaris, Calotropis procera, Calotropis procera, Melia azadarach, Chrysanthemum* spp., *Carica papaya, Heracleum* spp., *Azadirachta indica, Allium sativum, Heyysarvum coronarium, Artemisia maritime, etc.* showed potential anthelmintic activities against nematode parasites.

Immunological Approaches

Several natural antigens have been used to develop protection through vaccination but none have been mass produced. Vaccines have been developed to the "hidden" antigens and "natural" antigens. Hidden antigens are those which do not cause a detectable immune response in the host with natural infections and are thought to be internal antigens of the nematode. The first most effective vaccine against a GI parasites was Barbervax against *H. contortus*, release in October 2014. A "hidden" antigen vaccine Barbervax can be use for lambs, 5 subcutaneous injections of 1 ml, at approximately 6-week intervals (David Smith Moredun Research Institute, Edinburgh, UK). Some effective antigen which are under trial period are H11 (*H. contortus*), Tropomysin 41 (*Trichostrongylus columbriformis*) and ES31 (*Oestertagia circumcincta*) in sheep.

Biological Control

Bio-control agent's origin may be from plants like grasses, or from zoological origin like bacteria, fungus, virus, parasite and predator. Fungi that exhibit anti nematode properties have been known for a long time. They are divided into three major groups based on their morphology and types of nematode destroying properties. The first the group the predacious fungi produces specialized nematode-trapping structures (adhesive knobs, networks, rings *etc.*) on the mycelium. The species of predacious fungus which has received most attention recently is *Arthobotrys* spp. (*A. oligospora*) and *Monacrosporium* spp. The second group, the endoparasitic fungi, produce spores which either by penetration of cuticle from sticky spores adhering to the cuticle or following ingestion of spores which lodged in the gut. Examples of endoparasitic fungi are *Drechmeria coniospora* and *Harposporium anguillulae*. The third group the egg parasitic fungi have the ability to attack the egg stage and may have a role in the control of animal parasites which have a long development and/or survival time in the egg stage in the environment outside host. Eggs of *Ascaris lumbricoides* collected from naturally infected pigs were used mainly to test the effect of the fungus *Verticillium chlamydosporium* but also other *Verticillium* spp. the fungus was shown to be able to degrade the egg shell enzymatically and infect the eggs.

Nutritional Management

The strongest link between nutrition and parasitism has been illustrated between protein intake and resistance to GI nematode infection. Animals on low protein diets are more susceptible to infection because they produce less IgA (immunoglobulin). Minerals (Cu, Zn, Fe, Cobalt, phosphorus) and Vitamin supplements (A, B_{12}, E) amount a better immune response to internal parasites. Surprisingly, addition of molybdenum at 6-10 mg Mo/day decreased worm burdens in lambs that were not attributable to the expected copper deficiency. Molybdenum may have a role in increasing jejunal mast cells and blood eosinophils numbers.

Genetics Management

It is best long term weapon against internal parasites as some breeds are more resistant and resilient to internal parasites. Selection for parasite resistance breed is possible and will not adversely affect growth of animals. Recent years breeding policy has more concentrated on the development of parasites resistance breed. Parasites trait is moderately heritable 20-40 per cent. Grazing resistant breeds with susceptible breeds, may act to "sweep" pastures and reduce contamination to susceptible animals. Some breeds which are resistance against GI nematodes; Red Masai sheep, Florida Native Sheep, St. Croix Sheep, Galore and Barbados Back belly.

General Management

Parasite control starts with good management and common sense. Animal should not be fed on the ground. Water should be clean and free from faecal matter. Facilities of proper drainage in the anima shed reduce the chance of survival of the parasites, Pastures and pens should not be overstocked. When new animal are acquired they should be isolated from the rest of the flock for days and aggressively dewormed to prevent the introduction of drug-resistant worms.

1. Use of Clean or Safe Pastures

Safe pastures means the pasture which are not contaminated with the worm larvae and clean pastures means the pasture which are not been grazed by sheep or goats for the past 6 to 12 months but by horses or cattle. Hay or silage crop has been removed. Rotated with field crops. Burning a pasture will remove worm larvae.

2. Pasture Rest and Rotation

Resting period varied from 2 months (semiarid) to 6 months (cool moist climate) but 60- 65 day rest period is sufficient. In rotational grazing system ideally, sheep/goat should not be returned to the same pasture for 2-3 months.

3. Alternate Grazing System/Graze Multiple Species

Grazing between different age group of different species taking each species has different grazing behaviour that complements one another. Cattle/horse act as vacuum cleaner to the pasture if grazed before or after sheep/goat. Pastures grazed by cattle and horses are safer for sheep/goats (Area where *T. axei* is not a major problem). Sheep/goat does not graze together on same pasture.

4. Grazing Strategies

Stocking rate is an important consideration in parasite control as it affects exposure to infective larvae and contamination of the pasture. Thumb rules include 5–7 goats or 5 sheep being the equivalent of 1 cow, and suggestions of 5–7 goats/acre. Goats prefer to browse brush and trees, whereas sheep prefer to graze near the ground. Pasture management must include monitoring the condition of the herbage to ensure that overgrazing does not occur and to maintain a productive pasture.

5. Zero Grazing

Keeping animal in confinement (*i.e.* "zero grazing") is a means of reducing parasitism and preventing re-infection. Under a zero grazing situation, animal does not have access to any vegetation for grazing.

6. Use of Bioactive Forages

The pasture plants containing condensed tannins have anthelmintic properties. Condensed tannins (CT) are not only included in certain plants, a lot of plants have CT content but only those with higher levels are referred to as 'bioactive forage'. Some examples of bioactive forages are Chicory, Birdsfoot Trefoil, Sulla, Sainfoin, Quebracho *etc.*

7. Community Dilution

The only option that holds promise for practical application in the field is to engineer reversion by overwhelmingly diluting resistant worms with susceptible worm strains.

8. Refugia

It means the proportion of the worm population escaping exposure to anthelmintics. Most parasitologists now consider level of refugia as the single most important factor contributing to selection for anthelmintic resistance in parasites. The size of population in refugia at the time of anthelmintic treatment will determine the contribution of surviving worms to the subsequent generation and this was presented as a major source of resistance. Worms in refugia provides a pool of genes susceptible to anthelmintics, thus diluting the frequency of resistance genes. As the relative size of refugia increases, the rate of evolution towards resistance decreases. The density of parasite in refugia plays a major role in augmenting the rate of development of anthelmintic resistance.

Conclusion

Parasites are a major cause of disease and production loss in livestock, frequently causing significant economic loss and impacting on animal welfare. In addition to the impact on animal health and production, diagnosis and control measures are costly and often time-consuming. A major concern is the development of resistance by worm to many of chemical used to control them. Therefore is a urgent need for development of early detection methods along with planned preventive programs to minimize the risk of parasitic disease outbreak and sub clinical losses of animal production. Some techniques must be used such as smart drenching, FAMACHA, the five point check and increased housing management which can help to manage parasites. These techniques reduce dependence on dewormers and lead to a more sustainable parasite-management program. Integration of more than one measure like good farming practices, best breeding strategies, nutritional management, appropriate herbal anthelmintic, biological, immunological control measures, scientific utilization of biotechnological tools, mathematical models, decision support system and appropriate chemical control measures is essential to achieve the sustainable control on the parasites.

Chapter 6

Strategies for Management of Anthelmintic Resistance in Gastrointestinal Nematodes of Small Ruminants

C.P. Swarnkar

Division of Animal Health.
ICAR- Central Sheep and Wool Research Institute,
Avikanagar – 304501, Rajasthan
e-mail: swarnkarcp@yahoo.com

Among livestock, small ruminants play a big role in supporting the livelihood and proved to be life saviour in many distress conditions, especially in case of drought etc. for the rural poor livestock keepers. The productive potential of small ruminants is limited by several factors with parasitism as major one. In small ruminants, gastrointestinal nematodes (GINs) are common helminth parasites and the immune system keeps the worm burden at such levels that clinical symptoms usually do not occur. However, if this balance is not obtained or when intensity pressure is very high, GINs may severely impact the performance, production, reproduction and survival of host. The chronic nature of infection resulted in high morbidity and huge production losses in economic sense. An exhaustive review commissioned to prioritize animal health research for poverty reduction in the developing World, by an international donor consortium consisting of the WHO, OIE and FAO concluded that gastrointestinal parasitism had the highest global index as an animal health constraint to the poor. With partial farm budgeting approach, it was found that GINs with intensity of >500 epg during wormy season are responsible for causing an annual loss of Rs. 1491.71 and 341.13 million in adult and yearling sheep of Rajasthan, respectively. The overall annual loss was estimated to be Rs. 245.35 and Rs. 187.43 per adult and yearling sheep, respectively (Singh *et al.*, 2011). The overall economic loss due to GINs in sheep flocks of Rajasthan comprised of losses in mutton production (60.72 per cent), increased mortality (20.74 per cent) and premature culling (14.08 per cent), reduced fertility (4.10 per cent) and wool yield (0.36 per cent). The introduction of benzimidazole (BZ) anthelmintics in the 1960's led to a revolution in parasite control. By the 1970's and 80's new anthelmintic drug classes became available and rotation between drugs became a common practice. Since long for small ruminants, the standard parasite control measures in practice are:

- Frequent anthelmintic drench without considering intensity of infection, climate and grazing management
- En-mass deworming – ignoring the role of *refugia* in preservation of susceptibility in worm population
- Advocating and adopting dose and move strategy – Increased spread of anthelmintic resistant worms
- Frequent rotation of anthelmintic type

With this everyone thought they had seen the end of ill thrift due to the control of sub-clinical internal parasitism. But good things come to an end with various GI parasites developing resistance to anthelmintics *i.e.*, these drugs lose their effect within a decade. Thus, since centuries total or satisfactory control of GI parasitism could not be achieved. The existence of anthelmintic resistance (AR) came to light in the mid-1950s as a result of the failure of phenothiazine to control haemonchosis in a sheep flock in USA (Drudge *et al.*, 1957). The effectiveness of anthelmintics and the welfare and production benefits they bring are threatened by the increasing prevalence and severity of AR (Kaplan and Vidyashankar 2012). The emergence of anthelmintic resistance had a considerable impact on chemotherapeutic based worm management programmes. Farmers see their practical and easy way of worm control fading away, the pharmaceutical industry finds that the length of product life-cycles is reduced and veterinary practitioners lose an essential tool to use when providing advice on effective control programs. As a consequence, an escalation of anthelmintic resistance in parasite population resulted in hampering of all efforts employed to manage the problem of worms. The veterinary parasitology community is well aware of the threat posed by diminished efficacy of our most potent class of anthelmintics. However, these concerns cannot reach the producer until scientists and advisors develop a cohesive message about monitoring and management of worms and anthelmintic resistance in them.

Anthelmintic Resistance (AR)

It is defined as the ability of parasites to survive doses of drugs that would normally kill parasites of the same species and stage. It is a situation where a population of nematodes originally sensitive to anthelmintic, inherit the ability to survive treatment after repeated exposure to the drug (Sargison *et al.*, 2010; Torres-Acosta *et al.*, 2012). It has a genetic basis and may be either pre-adaptive (alleles conferring resistance may either be present in populations prior to drug exposure) or spontaneous (may occur *de novo* during the period of drug exposure). The resistance genes that occur through mutation are initially rare in the population but, as selection continues, the frequency of resistance genes increases and consequently the proportion of resistant parasites increases too. Anthelmintic resistance is multi-dimensional *i.e.* physiological or biological in property, genetic for inheritance, evolutionary for development of genetic strain and ecological for spread. The development of AR in worms is a multistage process and involving susceptible, intermediate and resistant phases (Figure 6.1).

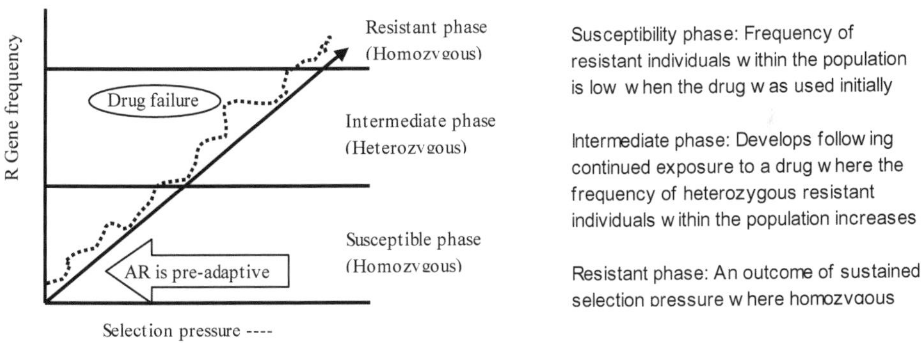

Figure 6.1: Intrinsic Phases in the Selection Process for Anthelmintic Resistance in Worms

The occurrence of AR came to light in the mid-1950s as a result of the failure of phenothiazine to control haemonchosis in a flock of sheep kept at a research farm in Kentucky, USA. The first report of decreased efficacy of TBZ against *H. contortus* strains dates from 1964, just 3 yrs after its introduction to the market (Drudge *et al.*, 1964). Similarly, resistance to imidazothiazole-tetrahydropyrimidine (Le Jambre *et al.*, 1976) and avermectin-milbemycin (Carmichael *et al.*, 1987) classes developed within 3-9 yrs after introduction to the market in sheep. Resistance to derquantel (Kaminsky *et al.*, 2011) and to monepantel (Scott *et al.*, 2013) has also been reported around the world, demonstrating the high vulnerability of these drugs. In India, although there is a lack of systematic monitoring of anthelmintic resistance, the country wide occurrence of resistance in GI nematodes against various classes of anthelmintics is evident through several scattered reports. Following the first report of AR in *H. contortus* to phenothiazine and thiabendazole in sheep at Pashulok, Rishikesh, U.P. (Varshney and Singh (1976), there were no documented reports of anthelmintic resistance till 1990. From 1990 onwards, there has been a renewed interest on this aspect and since then a considerable number of reports of anthelmintic resistance in GINs of small ruminants are pouring in from various parts of the country (Figures 6.2 and 6.3).

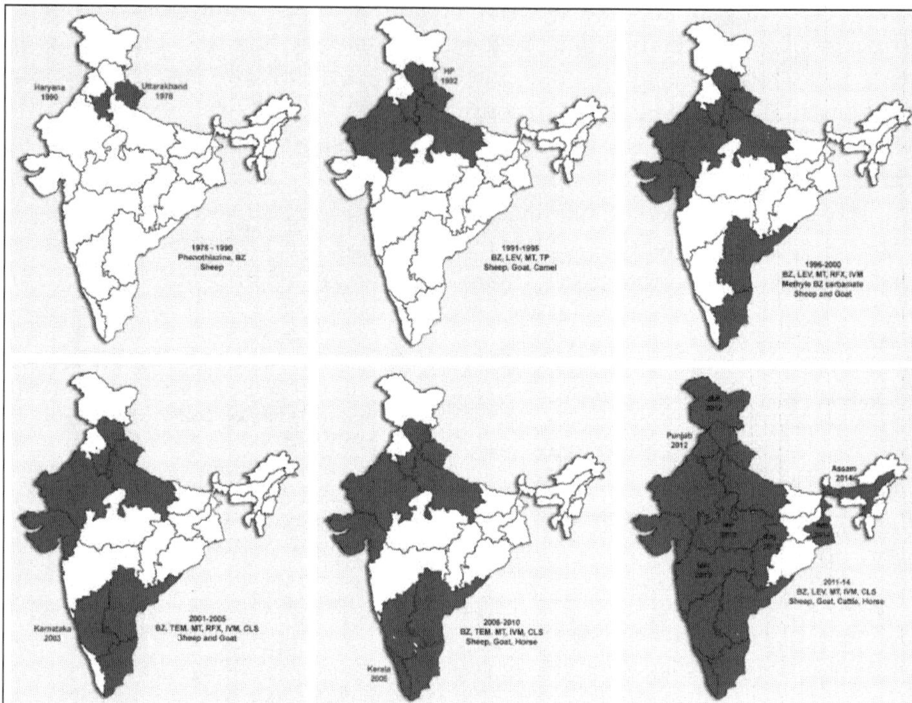

Figure 6.2: Progression of Anthelmintic Resistance in GI Nematodes of Livestock India

Mechanism of Anthelmintic Resistance

Anthelmintic resistance in nematodes is thought to be a pre-adaptive and multi-dimensional, arises from selection within the normal population. It is a physiological or biological property, its inheritance is genetical and development of genetic strain is evolutionary. The development of AR in worms is a multistage process consisting of susceptible (predominance of susceptible worms), intermediate (increase in the proportion of resistant larvae on the pasture) and resistant phase (predominance of resistance worms). Resistance in worms can be the result of a variety of mechanisms and can be roughly categorised as genetic changes in the drug target, changes in the drug transport or changes in the metabolism of the drug within the parasite (James *et al.*, 2007). F200Y (TAC) isotype-1 b-tubulin BZ resistance mutation is common in *H. contortus* throughout the world and the F167Y (TAC) and E198A (GCA) mutations, although less common, have been reported from different countries (Chaudhry

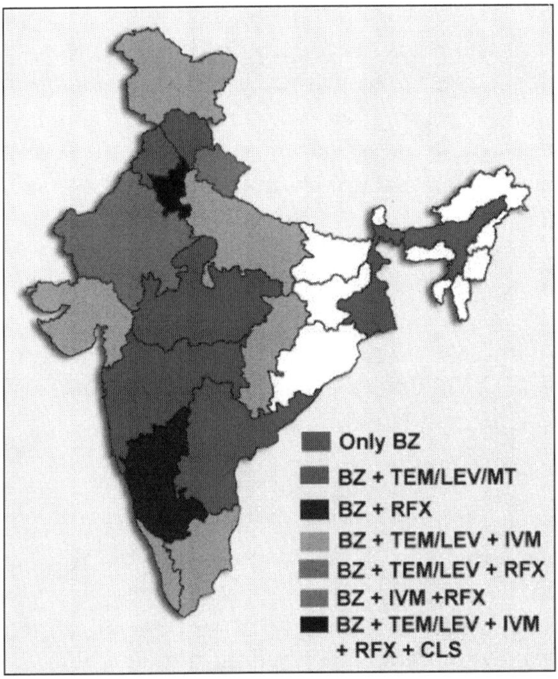

Figure 6.3: Anthelmintic-Wise Status of Anthelmintic Resistance in India

et al., 2015). In *H. contortus* populations from small ruminants across southern India, Chaudhry *et al.* (2015) mainly detected F200Y (TAC) mutation followed by E198A (GCA) mutation however not detected F167Y (TAC) mutation. Changes in drug transport mechanisms or in the metabolism of the drug within a worm species also account for different resistance mechanisms to the same anthelmintic (Vokral *et al.*, 2013). The P-glycoprotein, a cell membrane transport protein able to transport many different drugs may lead to multi drug resistance by increasing the active transport of drugs (Kerboeuf *et al.*, 2003). Riou *et al.* (2005) reported that the embryonation in *H. contortus* eggs induces a significant and gradual increase in egg shell fluidity which may be associated with an increased resistance to anthelmintics. The mechanism of resistance to LEV has not yet been fully elucidated. It is thought to be caused either by a reduction of the number of nicotinic acetylcholinesterase receptors or by a decreased affinity of these receptors for the drug. Blackhall *et al.* (1998) reported that one allele of the putative α-subunit gene is associated with resistance to the IVM. Therefore, more research is needed in order to understand the mechanisms and to develop suitable assays for detection of resistance.

Genetic Basis of Anthelmintic Resistance

The genetics of AR is complex as the number of genes involved and whether they are dominant or recessive, affects the rate at which resistance develops

(Leathwick *et al.*, 2001). Gene dominance refers to the ability of heterozygotes to survive a particular drug. If a drug kills the same high percentage of heterozygotes as the susceptible heterozygotes, the resistance gene is recessive. If the heterozygous genotype has equivalent ability to survive the resistant homozygote, the resistance gene is dominant. BZ resistance in *H. contortus* and *T. colubriformis* and other strongylids appears partly recessive trait (Dobson *et al.*, 1996). With *T. colubriformis,* LEV resistance is inherited as a sex-linked recessive trait, controlled either by a single gene or a cluster of tightly linked genes (Martin and McKenzie, 1990). In contrast LEV resistance in *H. contortus* is inherited as a recessive sex-linked trait (Dobson *et al.*, 1996). Resistance to IVM is inherited as a completely dominant trait in *H. contortus* and *O. circumcincta* (Le Jambre *et al.*, 2000; Leathwick *et al.*, 2001) and as a partially dominant trait in *T. colubriformis* (Gopal *et al.*, 1999).

Management of Anthelmintic Resistance

The veterinarians and farmers continue to follow decades old traditional approaches of parasite control, without considering the biological logic or medical rationale of such approaches. As an example, if a veterinarian found a animal in herd/flock to be suffering from a bacterial infection, he would perform a physical examination then would initiate a therapeutic plan based on that specific diagnosis and his/her clinical experience and knowledge. The therapeutic plan might include use of an antibiotic, but because it is well known that unnecessary antibiotic treatment will promote drug resistance in bacteria, the veterinarian would never consider treating the remaining animals in herd/flock that all appeared clinically normal. However, that same veterinarian would probably not hesitate to treat every animal in herd/flock with an anthelmintic, even though not a single animal is showing any signs of parasitic disease. The recipe-based treatment programmes based solely on the calendar without regard to the medical needs of individual animal, the biology of the parasites or efficacy of the drug against the target parasites can no longer be justified or recommended. The dramatic change in dynamics of parasites, climate and management practices indicate that our worm management strategies need to be refined to meet the present challenges by shifting the target stages from adult parasites in the host to pre-parasitic stages on the pasture. Given the wide regional variation that exists between sheep management systems and the different parasites that inhabit them, it is hardly surprising that there are no universally applicable "blueprint" approaches for management of GINs. Most studies on GI nematode ecology in livestock have concluded that climatic conditions play an important role in the survival and transmission of parasite eggs and larvae. Therefore, to be effective, worm management strategies should be based on a sound understanding of the epidemiology of parasite in both host and environment.

As the saying goes, "if you can't beat them, join them", we are never going to achieve eradication of worms. It is the anthelmintic resistant worms which are our major concern and we need to keep worms susceptible to the anthelmintics that we have, in order to have some control over them. So we need to think sideways and implement an additional strategy that will hinder the growth of the resistant worms in population. Since long, in worm control practice it has been recommended that all animals in a flock should be drenched with an anthelmintic at the same time. However, this strategy has turned out to be unsustainable and researchers now favour a selective approach where only those animals in need of anthelmintic intervention actually receive medication. This selective approach is highly compatible with host-parasite-environment interaction. Majority of parasitologists now considered levels of *refugia* as the single most important factor contributing to selection for anthelmintic resistance in parasites. Treating animals with low worm burdens does little to control parasites, but removes an important source of *refugia*, thereby accelerating the evaluation of resistance. Thus, consideration of double-edged problem in worms and their management is need of hour. There is a paradigm shift in the way to deal with parasites – away from flock control and the chemical 'big hit' approach to something more akin to parasite management *i.e.* "living with worms". The key areas of concern in the management of anthelmintic resistant nematodes throughout the world are:

- ✰ To limit its development on farm
- ✰ To limit its transmission by animals between farms
- ✰ On farm management of resistant populations

Results of various studies on anthelmintic resistance point towards the need for strategies aimed at delaying the onset of resistance. These strategies inevitably involve minimal chemoprophylaxis, minimizing the number of parasite generations exposed to a drug and also seek to maximize efficacy, thus effective rendering the genes for resistance recessive. Broadly, to reduce the need for anthelmintics and consequently to delay to development of resistance, the strategies are classified as anthelmintic based strategies, *refugia* based strategies and non-chemical strategies.

Anthelmintic Based Strategies

Anthelmintics

An anthelmintic is a substance that expels or destroys GI worms. Before 1940, the compounds used to deal with parasitism were the natural substances that had some effect on parasites, but also risked toxicity to the animal. The modern age of deworming began with the introduction of phenothiazine. In the 1960's and 70's, organophosphate anthelmintics were introduced but removed from the market due to toxicity issues. Now-a-days, anthelmintics are classified on the basis of similar chemical structure and mode of action as mentioned below:

Anthelmintic Class	*Mode of Action*
Benzimidazoles/ Probenzimidazole	Bind to β-tubulin and prevent the formation of microtubules. Interfere with the worm's energy metabolism on a cellular level. Causes the inhibition of glucose uptake, protein secretion and microtubule production, leading to starvation of the parasite.
Imidazothiazoles/ tetrahydropyrimidines	Mimic the action of acetylcholine causing depolarisation of nematode muscle bag membrane with an outflow of Na^+ leading to spastic paralysis of the worms.
Macrocyclic lactones (avermectins/milbemycins)	Act by opening of glutamate-gated chloride channels of neuromuscular membrane of nematodes with flaccid paralysis of the somatic musculature and inhibit feeding of adult worms.
Salicylanilides/Substituted Nitrophenols	Narrow spectrum proton ionopheres act by uncoupling the oxidative phosporylation leading to depletion of energy
Amino-acetonitrile derivatives (Monepantel)	Paralyzes worms by attacking a previously undiscovered receptor HCO-MPTL-1, present only in nematodes
Spiroindole (Derquantel)	It is a nicotinic cholinergic antagonist

Although anthelmintics are sold under several brand names, there are only a few chemical classes of dewormers. All drugs in a chemical class kill the worms in the same manner, though the effectiveness within chemical families varies. For drug rotation to be of any value, you need to switch chemical classes, not just brand name products.

Use of antelmintics is the only important control measure adopted throughout the world. These can be used either as curative or preventive. Curative application means use of anthelmintics on appearance of clinical manifestation of GIN. The disadvantages of curative control is that production losses already have occurred and the appearance of symptoms will often coincide with the presence of large populations of infective larvae on pasture, so we can usually expect immediate post-treatment reinfection. While using anthelmintics therapeutically, be ensure that, if the drug is not active against all stages, it must be effective against the pathogenic stages of the parasite, and after use of anthelmintic there should be a marked clinical improvement and rapid recovery. Preventive approach is aimed to reduce the contamination of pasture with parasite eggs, hence the rate of infection of sheep over some period in the future. The timing of treatment is based on the knowledge of epidemiology of GIN with reference to agro-climatic conditions. In general, four major forms of anthelmintic application are (i) conventional treatment, (ii) strategic treatment, (iii) targeted treatment and (iv) targeted selective treatment.

(i) ***Conventional treatment*** **(*CT*):** It is commonly practiced and consists of en-mass treatment with anthelmintics 2-4 times a year. The timings of treatment are either usually based on information in literatures/books *i.e.* without considering actual epidemiological profile in particular set of environment and management. The anthelmintic interventions are made at frequent interval as per availability money with farmer. A high frequency of treatments, indiscriminate use, en-mass treatment, prolonged use of single class of anthelmintics, under-dosing and use of anthelmintics during climatic extremes *etc.* lead to increased selection pressure in nematode populations and rampant rise in incidence of anthelmintic resistance.

(ii) ***Strategic treatment***: It consists of en-mass treatment of flock on the basis of historical knowledge of parasite epidemiology (eg. drenching at pre-monsoon, monsoon, post-monsoon, around lambing *etc.*). This practice was found to be costly and labour intensive along with responsible for severe increase in selection pressure for anthelmintic resistance, gradual decline in efficacy of anthelmintics and reduction in quantum of *refugia* (Swarnkar and Singh, 2013).

(iii) ***Targeted treatment (TT)*:** It involves treatment to whole flock at the most appropriate times bearing in mind the need to maintain *refugia*. These treatments differ from strategic treatments which are generally given prophylactically on the basis of epidemiology in a given area and are used to protect animals and prevent disease over a substantial period. To determine the most suitable time for anthelmintic intervention a thought needs to be given on bioclimatograph and rearing/grazing practices (Swarnkar and Singh, 2011). It serves to reduce the numbers of anthelmintic treatments and thus minimise pasture contamination with resistant genotypes. Effective targeting should also lead to an increased interval between treatments, allowing susceptible genotypes a better opportunity to establish on pasture and so reduce the risk of heterozygotes mating and producing homozygous resistant offspring. In Rajasthan, the experience gained after over the years by application of anthelmintic drench during mid to late monsoon showed increase in *refugia* with high efficacy of anthelmintics for prolonged period. The comparative evaluation of two schemes showed reduction in drench frequency in farm flocks had not hampered the flock productivity (Swarnkar and Singh, 2015). Like-wise in field flocks, annual lambing, purchase, sale and morbidity rates were remained almost similar in both the categories of flocks. However, annual mortality rate was slightly higher (10.01 per cent) in CT flocks compared to 7.98 per cent in TT flocks (Singh *et al.*, 2018).

Over dispersion in faecal egg counts: Assumption like that each host is infected with the same number of worms should not be a criterion for *en-mass* anthelmintic intervention as GINs in small ruminants are highly over-dispersed, with around 80 per cent of the worms found in only 20-30 per cent of the host (Hoste *et al.*, 2001). Studies showed that during favourable season (Jul-Sep) around 20-30 per cent and 50 per cent of sheep in field and farm conditions, respectively had FECs to the tune of >1000 epg (Singh *et al.*, 2018). In recent times, it has been recognized that the phenomenon of parasite over-dispersion could be put to good use if those animals suffering from level of infection sufficient to cause considerable production loss or health effects, can be identified and treated individually. This phenomenon can be used in form of targeted selective treatment (TST) and for breeding for resistance/resilience to parasites (Malan *et al.*, 2001). By adopting this practice not only the cost of anthelmintic and labour will be reduced, but the proportions of worms in *refugia* will be greatly increased as the untreated animals – usually the majority – will be voiding eggs from unselected worms, compared to the few eggs from effectively dewormed animals.

(iv) ***Targeted selective treatment* (*TST*)**: Following prioritized *H. contortus* as major nematode species of economic importance in small ruminants and occurrence of over-dispersion phenomenon in FECs, a technique was standardized to identify those animals in flock which harbour higher intensity of infection, suffer with clinical form of diseases and are actually in need of chemotherapeutic intervention. TST is a method of identifying heavily parasitized individual animal, based on physical evidence of anaemia caused by *H. contortus*. TST is directed towards those animals that are susceptible or that most contaminate pasture and this requires the ability to identify these individuals within a flock. A colour chart based on ocular mucous membrane, microhaematocrit and intensity of infection in sheep was developed and tested at ICARI-CSWRI, Avikanagar. With TST application it was observed that frequency of anthelmintic treatment/year ranged from 8.65 per cent to 29.31 per cent an average of 16.80 per cent compared to >100 per cent drenching in CT/TT approach. The application of TST is feasible and effective not only in managing the haemonchosis but also help in increasing the size of *refugia* which may ultimately resulted into both maintenance of drug efficacy against parasites and sizeable reduction in the cost of worm management in sheep flocks. The main disadvantages are the difficulty and time spent on selecting animals in need of treatment and the possibility of lower production. The comparative evaluation of TT and TST showed that in monetary terms the net annual income/100 sheep remained higher (Rs. 53024.00) in flock managed for worms with TST approach with use of anthelmintic at a frequency of 0.13 drench/head/annum compared to a net annual income of Rs. 37448.00 in flocks where GIN infection was managed with TT approach with use of anthelmintics at the frequency of 1.61 drench/head/annum. This method also serves as a good tool to identify sheep that repeatedly require anthelmintic intervention so

that such animals may be culled from the flock. However there still a need for cheap, reliable diagnostic technique to identify individual animal needing treatment, where other species like *Trichostrongylus, Oesophagostomum* etc. predominates (Singh and Swarnkar, 2012; Swarnkar and Singh, 2014).

Smart Drenching

The term "Smart Drenching" was coined to describe selective treatment of certain animals with the goal to maintain animal health and production while decreasing the rate of development of parasite resistance to anthelmintics (Singh *et al.*, 2015). It encourages producers to use anthelmintics selectively, judiciously and effectively. It involves:

- ☆ Identification of effective anthelmintic type in an area through faecal egg count reduction test
- ☆ Proper dose calculation (based on maximum body weight in similar age-group of animals)
- ☆ Ensure administration of correct amount of over the animal's tongue and to the back of its throat
- ☆ Use dewormers from two different classes if resistance is suspected on the farm
- ☆ Keep animals to be wormed off feed for 12-24 hours before treating with benzimidazoles or ivermectin, doramectrin and moxidectin
- ☆ Only deworm animals that require treatment. Use the conjunctiva colour chart to assess animals with clinical anaemia due to *H. contortus*. For other parasites, base treatment on body condition, age, faecal egg count, performance/production, pregnancy/lactation status, signs and short-term weight gain

The benefits of smart drenching are 3-fold – (i) reduced cost of worm management as fewer animals (maximum of 20-30 per cent during wormy season) are dewormed, (ii) reduced selection pressure on parasites to develop resistance and (iii) preservation of anthelmintic efficacy for prolonged period due to increased quantum of *refugia.*

Refugia Based Strategies

"The solution to pollution is dilution."*Refugia* can simply be defined as a population that is either unexposed to or, in certain circumstances, unaffected by an anthelmintic. All the three components of host-parasite-environment triod plays crucial role in maintaining the quantum of *refugia*. Worms in *refugia* provides a pool of genes susceptible to anthelmintics, thus diluting the frequency of resistance genes (van Wyk, 1990). Appropriate treatment strategies and pasture management need to be implemented to maintain *refugia*. The parasite based approaches are based on the frequency of the resistant alleles in the parasite population, the biotic potential of the parasite and the longevity of both the supra- and infra-populations (Fleming *et al.*, 2006; Graef *et al.*, 2013; van Wyk, 2001). The frequency of resistant genes influences the rate at which homozygous resistant parasites appear in the population. If the proportion of resistance genes is high, then there is an increased probability that heterozygotes will have the opportunity to mate and produce homozygous resistant offspring. The degree of biotic potential of a parasite species determines the numbers of individuals of that species required to provide a given level of *refugia*. For example, species with high biotic potential, *e.g. H. contortus*, can provide a high degree of pasture contamination from relatively few individuals and therefore, effective *refugia* can, assuming successful completion of the lifecycle, be maintained by leaving a relatively small proportion of the host population unexposed to treatment. In other species with lower biotic potential, *e.g. Trichostrongylus* spp., a greater proportion of the host population would need to be left unexposed to treatment to provide the same level of *refugia*. A study conducted at ICAR-CSWRI, Avikanagar on the seasonal variation in different genotypes of *H. contortus* exhibited that sheep harbour more number of BZ-susceptible worms during monsoon and winter compared to summer. The relatively higher proportion of rr genotype in supra-population during the period from March to July indicates existence of unsuitable climate for larval dissemination as well as meagre chances of re-infection from pasture (Swarnkar *et al.*, 2012). The concept of *refugia* can be applied to slow the development of anthelmintic resistance through the use of approaches such as dilution of resistant with susceptible parasites when the proportion of resistance alleles is high, and targeted and selectively targeted treatments when resistant alleles are less common.

Community Dilution Strategy

The only option that holds promise for practical application in the field is to engineer reversion by overwhelmingly diluting resistant worms with susceptible worm strains. An entirely different approach to the management of resistance has been attempted in South Africa where an attempt has been made to reintroduce susceptible gene in to the *supra population*. Similarly, while working with sheep flocks of State Sheep Breeding Farm, Fatehpur (Rajasthan), it was experienced that community dilution strategy help in reversion to susceptibility for BZ. In this farm BZ resistance was first confirmed in 1998 using FECRT with 0.00 per cent efficacy for benzimidazole anthelmintics. On subsequent years there was gradual rise in per cent FECR whenever examined and with marginal rise in BZ susceptible alleles. On exploration the causes of these findings it was found that unwanted introduction of field animals infected with BZ susceptible strains of *H. contortus* for grazing on pasture area of farm leads to dilution of resistant population in refugia with resultant increase in anthelmintic efficacy at farm. The correlated response between genotypic frequency of homozygous BZ-resistant larvae and BZ-efficacy exhibited that a marginal rise in the proportion of BZ-susceptible alleles during September to November resulted in increase in efficacy of BZ anthelmintics as well as reduces the proportion of flocks harbouring BZ-resistant *H. contortus*. The period from September to November in semi-arid and from June to February in arid Rajasthan was found appropriate in increasing the frequency of BZ-susceptible alleles in the *refugia* (Swarnkar *et al.*, 2012; Singh and Swarnkar, 2017; Swarnkar *et al.*, 2021). Although this approach has the potential to reduce the prevalence of resistant parasites on a given area, there are practical limitations which may prevent its widespread use, *e.g.* the availability of large numbers of pathogen-free susceptible larvae with which to infect seeder animals and the ability to reduce pasture contamination to negligible levels.

Breeding for Increasing Resistance/Resilience to GINs

Animals can minimize the detrimental impact of parasites in two ways, firstly by limiting the number of parasites (resistance) and secondly, by reducing their impact on production (resilience). The largest source of genetic variation in resistance is between sheep within a flock, rather than between different flocks (Bisset *et al.*, 2001). In most studies, FEC was the main phenotypic measurement used for selection of the responding animals. The heritability of resistance to GIN infection in sheep, as measured by FEC varied from 0.01 to 0.50 (Prince *et al.*, 2010; Gowane *et al.*, 2019). Using FEC as phenotypic marker for within breed selection of resistant and/or susceptible animals at ICAR-CSWRI, Avikanagar, it was observed that this trait is low to moderately heritable. The profile of intensity of strongyle infection in divergent lines (resistant "R" and susceptible "S") over the years exhibited that animals of R-line had lower monthly FECs compared to their counterparts in S-line. The animals of S-line required strategic as well as tactical anthelmintic intervention while animals of R-line were maintained without any anthelmintic intervention (Singh *et al.*, 2009; Swarnkar *et al.*, 2009; Gowane *et al.*, 2020). In addition, the reduced worm egg production by worm resistant sheep will have a favourable epidemiological effect by decreasing the infectivity of pastures by worm larvae.

Management Based Strategies

Following management practices are advocated to manage gastrointestinal nematodes and to delay the anthelmintic resistance in them:

Avoid Treatment on Low-Contaminated Pastures

The most recognized high risk practice today is the use of anthelmintic treatments associated with pastures carrying low numbers of susceptible nematode larvae (van Wyk, 2001). As the rate of reinfection post-treatment is slow, the surviving worms remain undiluted by new infection for a protracted period. In areas where dry summer conditions result in almost no survival of nematode larvae on pasture, drenching during summer is highly selective for resistance (Swarnkar and Singh, 2010; Woodgate and Besier, 2010).

Check for Peri-parturient Rise in FECs

Anthelmintic treatment of adult ewes around lambing has been a common practice for many years and this select for anthelmintic resistance. The epidemiological studies at several places indicated absence of typical rise in feacal egg counts around lambing. Therefore, assessment of peri-parturient rise in worm egg count need to established in given agroclimatic condition and based on findings, climate and grazing resources, worm management programme should be modified. The absence of this phenomenon resulted in successful withdrawal of anthelmintic drench around parturition in sheep and goat flocks of Rajasthan (Swarnkar *et al.*, 1998; Singh and Swarnkar 2013; Choudhary *et al.*, 2021). This help in increased survival of susceptible parasites with in the host (as hypobiotic), reduced selection pressure for AR and maintain the efficacy of anthelmintics by increasing the size of *refugia*.

Avoid Dose and move Strategy

During 1970's, this strategy was central to the maintenance of clean grazing. Sheep were treated as they were moved on to clean pasture to prevent contamination. Unfortunately this practice is highly selective for anthelmintic resistance. Farming practices such as "drench-and-move" may provide a survival advantage for resistant parasites. The odds of having anthelmintic resistance were 4-times higher on farms that practiced drench and move, compared to those farms that did not, suggesting that this practice should be discouraged. When the dewormed animals are managed on the contaminated environment, new parasite populations in *refugia* rapidly gaining access into the host animal will continue to dilute the resistant sub-population that was selected by treatment in the animal body.

Prevent Introduction/Borrowing of Resistant Nematodes

As the prevalence of resistance has increased around the world, so too has the probability that animals transferred between farms will introduce anthelmintic resistant worms. In a premise anthelmintic resistant strain of parasites can introduced through selection by frequent treatment, through purchase of animals carrying resistant worms or through borrowing of strains from flocks grazed together on common property resources (Besier and Love, 2012). It was observed that use of both BZ and LEV groups of anthelmintics is common in field flocks of the same locality and worm population in *refugia* as well as in host was comprised of both susceptible and resistant to them. The flocks in which BZ was never used showed high prevalence of BZ resistant strains of parasite *vis- a- vis* flocks never drenched with LEV revealed prevalence of LEV resistance strains of parasites due to borrowing of strains from flocks grazed together on common property resources (Swarnkar and Singh, 2012). Effective management strategies to prevent development of anthelmintic resistance are worthless if producers purchase resistant worms residing in animals. "Quarantine" treatments for introduced stock have been widely advocated with the aim of completely removing the worm burden.

Grazing Management

It is stated that "Drenching is not a substitute for good feeding" and "There is no better anthelmintic than good quality green grass". The role of grazing management in worm control programme is simply to provide "low risk" pastures for the most susceptible sheep with the aim to provide better nutrition at the same time. It is most successful if applied when larval numbers are at low levels (Charlier *et al.*, 2010).

Rotational Grazing

The grazing system for livestock as followed by farmers is rotational in nature depending upon the availability of fodder. It has been observed that farmers put their animals on community grazing land/forest with the onset of monsoon where animals are drenched during mid-monsoon and continued on the same up to October. After harvesting of kharif crop the flocks are moved on such field to utilize crop stubbles for a period of one month. From November onward the flocks were again moved to community grazing land, forest or maintained on top feed with intermittent grazing on crop stubbles after rabi harvesting (Swarnkar *et al.*, 2008b).

Pasture Resting

It consists of preventing the animals from grazing in the same field or paddock. Since too low or too high temperature kill the infective larvae, cold and dry (hot dry) period can be relied upon to reduce or extend rest periods. In semi-arid conditions at least 2 month resting is essential compared to 6 month in cool, moist environment. In semi-arid Rajasthan, study with tracer lambs exhibited that sheep grazed during monsoon on spring contaminated-summer un-grazed pasture had very low FEC and worm count compared to those placed on continuously grazed contaminated pasture. The pasture larval burden was higher in general pasture than summer un-grazed pasture. Thus, resting the contaminated pasture during summer found to effectively control the pasture larval burden (Singh *et al.*, 1997; Swarnkar *et al.*, 1997).

In addition, other non-chemical practices are (i) allow to graze sheep flock on pasture >3″ in height due to abundance of infective strongyle larvae in water droplets on grass blades in the lower 3″ of forage, (ii) follow the Gumboot rule – avoid grazing on pasture with height shorter than the toe of gumboot, (iii) avoid grazing of flock on wet pastures, (iv) rotate pastures and allow as much rest time as possible between re-grazing (at least 6-9 weeks), (v) encourage practice of multi-species grazing, (vi) do not overstock animals on grazing area and (vii) encourage feeding of condensed tannin rich fodder.

Manure Treatment and Use of Fertilizers

Manure to be used for spreading may be filled with parasite eggs and larvae. Composting is a good way to clean manure as the eggs and larvae of nematode are killed at temperature as low as 32 to 34 °C. They are killed within 1 hr at 50 °C and in less than 4 hr at 44 °C. A few documented studies have shown that ammonium nitrate and other fertilizers as having larvicidal and ovicidal properties On pasture plots experimentally contaminated with eggs of the *H. contortus*, the translation from eggs to larvae was only 19.7 per cent following application of urea at a concentration of 1.25g N_2 per cent (corresponding to 27.17 Kg Urea/ha) compared to 100 per cent on untreated pasture plots (Swarnkar *et al.*, 2002).

Improve Host Nutrition

Several studies have brought evidence showing that manipulation of the host nutrition could represent an option to improve the host resistance and or resilience to parasites. The strongest link between nutrition and parasitism has been illustrated between protein intake and resistance to GIN infection. The most dramatic has been abolishment of the peri-parturient egg increase in lambing ewes by providing protein at 130 per cent of requirements. Incorporation of fodder containing condensed tannin in ruminant nutrition further reduces the dependence on anthelmintics by masking or diluting the pathogenic effects of worms (Swarnkar *et al.*, 2008a). Supplementation with phosphorus has been shown to prevent worm establishment. Treatment of lambs with copper oxide wires orally found to reduced *H. contortus* burdens. The addition of molybdenum (@ 6-10 mg/day) found to reduce the worm burdens in lambs (Sykes and Coop, 2001).

Biological Control

With in the environment the pre-parasitic stages of nematodes are subjected to a variety of both abiotic and biotic factors that can influence their development and survival. The abiotic factors are temperature, humidity and oxygen. Biotic factors comprised of vast assemblage of living organisms that can affect the success of worm eggs developing to infective larvae. BC agents rarely eliminate the target organism, but reduce their number to acceptable level and maintain a balance between the pathogen and the antagonist. Thus, BC may be defined as "an ecological method designed by man to lower a pest/parasite population to acceptable sub-clinical densities or to keep these populations at a non-pathogenic level using natural antagonists" (Khan *et al.*, 2001).

Monitoring and Planning Systems

Faecal Egg Count

Regular monitoring of FECs from flocks will help to indicate when dosing is really needed and equally important when it can be delayed or even omitted.

Faecal Egg Count Reduction Test

Only by knowing exactly the status of anthelmintic resistance in a farm, an appropriate action is taken. Otherwise using an ineffective or partly effective drug is not only a waste of money, but may also augment the resistant problem.

Use of Expert

Only knowledgeable Veterinarians, who are familiar with the area, farming system and risks, can construct a simple, practical, economic and effective strategy for worm control.

Use a Programme

Unless a planned system is in place and is used properly, the results will inevitably be seen. If based on ad-hoc decisions and the animals are either dosed too often or with inappropriate drug or at the wrong time or with no coherent plan yield no results. Thought out by setting up a well deworming plan, the number of ineffective doses can be reduced. This is one of the area in which the knowledge and skills of local Veterinarians are vital for its success.

Flexibility

The programme should be flexible to allow for changes in weather, management and farming systems, drug costs and other factors.

Conclusion

Internal parasites continue to be a threat to health and productivity of small ruminants. The parasites of major concern were *Haemonchus, Trichostrongylus* and *Oesophagostomum* throughout the country. Management of GINs presents a difficult challenge following wide-spread emergence of anthelmintic resistance and is further complicated by recent and radical changes in approach to worm management. A rising trend in rate of anthelmintic resistance has threatened the efficacy of valuable non-renewable anthelmintics and making chemical based worm management programme an un-sustainable option. Currently, there are no country-wide programmes that systematically monitor the occurrence of resistance in parasites of small ruminants. There must be regional worm control programmes based on detailed epidemiological and ecological studies of nematode infections of livestock in a variety of locations/ agro-climatic conditions. These programmes should include time and type of anthelmintic to be used, rotation of anthelmintic, if required, monitoring the efficacy of anthelmintic used and economic assessment of a control programme. Anthelmintic intervention in flocks should be restricted to the active parasite transmission season. Thus, we need to look at anthelmintics, not as a tool in our tool box, but as a band aid to fix a management problem. It is need of hour to promote targeted selective treatment at least at farm level. The alternate approaches in worm management need to be researched which require basic data to convince the policy planner for research fund aid to show the benefit to the farmers in adopting the technologies evolved with minimal use of chemotherapeutics.

REFERENCES

Besier RB and Love SCJ. 2012. Advising on helminth control in sheep: it's the way we tell them. *Vet. J.*, 193: 2-3.

Bisset SA, Morris CA, McEwan JC and Vlassoff A. 2001. Breeding sheep in New Zealand that are less reliant on anthelmintics to maintain health and productivity. *New Zealand Vet. J.*, 49: 236-246.

Blackhall WJ, Liu HY, Xu M, Prichard RK and Beech RN. 1998. Selection at a P-glycoprotein gene in ivermectin- and moxidectin-selected strains of *Haemonchus contortus*. Mol. Biochem. *Parasitol.*, 95: 193-201.

Carmichael I, Visser R, Schneider D and Soll M. 1987. *Haemonchus contortus* resistant to ivermectin. *J. S. Afr. Vet. Assoc.* 58: 93.

Charlier J, Demeler J, Hoglund J, von Samson-Himmelstjerna G, Dorny P and Vercruysse J. 2010. *Ostertagia ostertagi* in first-season grazing cattle in Belgium, Germany and Sweden: general levels of infection and related management practices. *Vet. Parasitol.*, 171: 91-98.

Chaudhary U, Rathore B and Swarnkar CP. 2021. Studies on peri-parturient rise phenomenon in faecal egg counts of goats in Jaipur district of semi-arid Rajasthan. *J. Vet. Parasitol.*, 35: 42-47.

Chaudhry U, Redman EM, Raman M and Gilleard JS. 2015. Genetic evidence for the spread of a benzimidazole resistance mutation across southern India from a single origin in the parasitic nematode *Haemonchus contortus*. *Int. J. Parasitol.*, 45: 721-728.

Dobson RJ, Le Jambre L and Gill JH. 1996. Management of anthelmintic resistance: inheritance of resistance and selection with persistent drugs. *Int. J. Parasitol.*, 26: 993-1000.

Drudge JH, Leland SE and Wyant ZN. 1957. Strain variation in the response of sheep nematodes to the action of phenothiazine. I. Studies of mixed infections in experimental animals. *Am. J. Vet. Res.*, 18: 133-341.

Drudge JH, Szanto J, Wyant ZN and Elam G. 1964. Field studies on parasite control in sheep: Comparison of thiabendazole, ruelene, and phenothiazine. *Am. J. Vet. Res.*, 25: 1512-1518.

Fleming SA, Craig T, Kaplan RM, Miller JE, Navarre C and Rings M. 2006. Anthelmintic resistance of gastrointestinal parasites in small ruminants. *J. Vet. Intern. Med.*, 20: 435-444.

Gopal RM, Pomray WE and West DM. 1999. Resistance of field isolates of *Trichostrongylus colubriformis* and *Ostertagia circumcincta* to ivermectin. *Int. J. Parasitol.*, 29: 781-786.

Gowane GR, Swarnkar CP, Misra SS, Kumar R, Kumar A and Prince LLL. 2019. Genetic parameter estimates for fecal egg counts and their relationship with growth in Avikalin and Malpura sheep. *Animal*, 13: 1788-1796

Gowane GR, Swarnkar CP, Misra SS, Kumar R, Kumar A, Singh D and Prince LLL. 2020. Selecting sheep for *Haemonchus contortus* resistance and susceptibility: flock dynamics and genetic architecture. *Res. Vet. Sci.*, 132: 116-126.

Graef J de, Claerebout E and Geldhof P. 2013. Anthelmintic resistance of gastrointestinal cattle nematodes. *Vlaams Diergeneeskundig Tijdschrift*, 82: 113-123.

Hoste H, Lefrileux Y and Pommaret A. 2001. Distribution and repeatability of faecal egg counts and blood parameters in dairy goats naturally infected with gastrointestinal nematodes. *Res. Vet. Sci.*, 70: 57-60.

James CE, Hudson AL and Davey MW. 2007. Drug resistance mechanisms in helminths: is it survival of the fittest? *Trends Parasitol.*, 25: 328-335.

Kaminsky R, Bapst B, Stein PA, Strehlau GA, Allan BA, Hosking BC, Rolfe PF and Sager H. 2011. Differences in efficacy of monepantel, derquantel and abamectin against multi-resistant nematodes of sheep. *Parasitol. Res.*, 109: 19-23.

Kaplan RM and Vidyashankar AN. 2012. An inconvenient truth: Globalworming and anthelmintic resistance. *Vet. Parasitol.*, 186: 70-78.

Kerboeuf D, Blackhalls W, Kaminskyc R and von Samson-Himmelstjernaa G. 2003. P-glycoprotein in helminths: function and perspectives for anthelmintic treatment and reversal of resistance. Efflux pumps and antibiotic resistance of microorganisms. *Int. J. Antimicrobial Agents*, 22: 332–346.

Khan FA, Swarnkar CP, Singh D, Bhagwan PSK and Dubey SC. 2001. Nematophagus fungi isolated from sheep faeces: a promising biological control of *Haemonchus contortus*. *Indian J. Anim. Sci.*, 71: 834-836

Le Jambre LF, Gill JH, Lenane IJ and Baker P. 2000. Inheritance of avermecin resistance in *Haemonchus contortus*. *Int. J. Parasitol.*, 30: 105-111.

Le Jambre LF, Southcott WH and Dash KM. 1976. Resistance of selected lines of *Haemonchus contortus* to thiabendazole, morantel tartrate and levamisole. *Int. J. Parasitol.*, 6: 217-222.

Leathwick DM, Pomroy WE and Heath ACG. 2001. Anthelmintic resistance in New Zealand. *New Zealand Vet. J.*, 49: 227-235.

Malan FS, van Wyk JA and Wessels CD. 2001. Clinical evaluation of anaemia in sheep : early trials. *Onderstepoort J. Vet. Res.*, 61: 165-174.

Martin PJ and McKenzie JA. 1990. Levamisole resistance in *Trichostrongylus colubriformis* : a sex-linked recessive character. *Int. J. Parasitol.*, 20: 867- 872.

Prince LLL, Gowane GR, Swarnkar CP, Singh D and Arora AL. 2010. Estimates of genetic parameters for faecal egg count of *Haemonchus contortus* infection and relationship with growth traits in Avikalin sheep. *Trop. Anim. Hlth Prod.*, 42: 785-791.

Riou M, Koch LM and Kerboeuf D. 2005. Increased resistance to anthelmintics of *Haemonchus contortus* eggs associated with changes in membrane fluidity of eggshells during embryonation. *Parasitol. Res.*, 95: 266-272.

Sargison ND, Jackson F, Wilson DJ, Bartley DJ, Penny CD and Gilleard J. 2010. Characterisation of milbemycin, avermectin, imidazothiazole and benzimidazole resistant *Teladorsagia circumcincta* from a sheep flock. *Vet. Rec.*, 166: 681-686.

Scott I, Pomroy WE, Kenyon PR, Smith G, Adlington B and Moss A. 2013. Lack of efficacy of monepantel against *Teladorsagia circumcincta* and *Trichostrongylus colubriformis*. *Vet. Parasitol.*, 196: 166-171.

Singh D and Swarnkar CP. 2012. Evaluation of targeted selective treatment strategy in sheep farm of Rajasthan. *Indian J. Anim. Sci.*, 82: 679-686.

Singh D and Swarnkar CP. 2013. Comparative impact of conventional and strategic worm management schemes in sheep flocks of arid Rajasthan. *Indian J. Anim. Sci.*,83: 1128-1134.

Singh D and Swarnkar CP. 2017. Worm control approaches and their impact on status of anthelmintic resistance at an organized sheep farm. *Indian J. Anim. Sci.*, 87: 568-572.

Singh D, Swarnkar CP and Khan FA. 2018. Epidemiology of gastrointestinal parasites and impact of worm management schemes in sheep flocks of Rajasthan. *Small Rumin. Res.*, 164: 22-27.

Singh D, Swarnkar CP and Sanyal PK. 2015. Dynamics of epidemiological intelligence for exploitation in effective worm management in sheep – A Rajasthan experience. *Indian J. Anim. Sci.*, 85: 679-694.

Singh D, Swarnkar CP, Khan FA, Srivastava CP and Bhagwan PSK. 1997. Epidemiology of ovine gastrointestinal nematodes at an organised farm in Rajasthan, India. *Small Ruminant Res.*, 26: 31-37.

Singh D, Swarnkar CP, Kumar Sushil, Prince LLL and Arora AL. 2009. Performance of Avikalin sheep selected for resistance to *Haemonchus contortus*. *J. Vet. Parasitol.*, 23: 23-27.

Singh D, Swarnkar CP, Prince LLL and Pathak, KML. 2011. Economic Analysis and Impact of Gastrointestinal Nematodes on Sheep Production in Rajasthan. Directorate of Knowledge Management in Agriculture, Indian Council of Agricultural Research, New Delhi, pp 1-84.

Swarnkar CP and Singh D. 2010. Worm control practices, anthelmintic use and its implication on anthelmintic resistance in gastrointestinal nematodes of sheep in Rajasthan. *Indian J. Anim. Sci.*, 80: 593-600.

Swarnkar CP and Singh D. 2011. Role of bioclimatographs in forecasting of strongyle infection in Rajasthan. *Indian J. Anim. Sci.*, 81: 216-223.

Swarnkar CP and Singh D. 2012. Role of quarantine in management of anthelmintic resistance in strongyle worms of sheep. *Indian J. Small Rumin.*, 8: 95-99.

Singh D and Swarnkar CP. 2013. Comparative impact of conventional and strategic worm management schemes in sheep flocks of arid Rajasthan. *Indian J. Anim. Sci.*, 83: 1128-1134.

Swarnkar CP and Singh D. 2014. Sensitivity and specificity analysis for targeted selective treatment using eye colour chart in sheep flocks naturally infected with *Haemonchus contortus* in Rajasthan. *Indian J. Anim. Sci.*, 84: 1177-1180

Swarnkar CP and Singh D. 2015. Epidemiology of ovine gastrointestinal parasites under different worm management strategies at an organized farm in arid Rajasthan. *Indian J. Small Rumin.*, 21: 53-63.

Swarnkar CP, Khan FA, Singh D, Sharma SR and Bhagwan PSK. 1998. Some observations on periparturient rise in ewes at an organised farm. *Indian Vet. J.*, 75: 781-784.

Swarnkar CP, Singh D and Kumar S. 2012. Prevalence of benzimidazole resistant β-tubulin alleles in *Haemonchus contortus* larvae from sheep of Rajasthan. *Indian J. Anim. Sci.*, 82: 1477-1481.

Swarnkar CP, Singh D, Khan FA and Sharma SR. 2021. Reversion towards benzimidazole susceptibility in *Haemonchus contortus* by resistance management strategies at an organized sheep farm in semi-arid Rajasthan. *Indian J. Anim. Sci.*, 91: 196-199.

Swarnkar CP, Singh D, Khan FA and Vaithiyanathan S. 2008a. Effect of tanniferous plant (*Prosopis cineraria*) on *Haemonchus contortus* infection in sheep. *Indian J. Anim. Sci.*, 78: 953-955.

Swarnkar CP, Singh D, Khan FA, Bhagwan PSK and Dubey SC. 2002. Effect of urea application on pre-parasitic stages of *Haemonchus contortus* and its role in reducing pasture infectivity. *J. Vet. Parasitol.*, 16: 23-26.

Swarnkar CP, Singh D, Khan FA, Srivastava CP and Bhagwan PSK. 1997. Development and survival of *Haemonchus contortus* larvae on pasture under semi-arid conditions of Rajasthan. *J. Vet. Parasitol.*, 11: 37-41.

Swarnkar CP, Singh D, Krishna Lal and Khan FA. 2008b. Epidemiology and Management of Gastrointestinal Parasites of Sheep flocks in Rajasthan. CSWRI, Avikanagar pp. 1 – 145

Swarnkar CP, Singh D. Kumar Sushil, Mishra AK and Arora AL. 2009. Study on Malpura sheep selected for resistance to *Haemonchus contortus*. *Indian J. Anim. Sci.*, 79: 577-581

Sykes AR and Coop RL. 2001. Interaction between nutrition and gastrointestinal parasitism in sheep. *New Zealand Vet. J.*, 49: 222-226.

Torres-Acosta JF, Mendoza-de-Gives P, Aguilar-Caballero AJ and Cuellar-Ordaz JA. 2012. Anthelmintic resistance in sheep farms: Update of the situation in the American continent. *Vet. Parasitol.*, 189: 89-96.

van Wyk JA. 1990. Integrated worm control as a strategy in the control of gastrointestinal nematodes of sheep and cattle. *J. S. Afr. Vet. Assoc.* 61: 141-145.

van Wyk JA. 2001. Refugia - Overlooked as perhaps the most potent factor concerning the development of anthelmintic resistance. *Onderstepoort J. Vet. Res.*, 68: 55-67.

Varshney TR and Singh YP. 1976. A note on development of resistance of *Haemonchus contortus* worms against phenothiazine and thiabendazole in sheep. *Indian J. Anim. Sci.*, 46: 666-668.

Vokral I, Jirasko R, Stuchlikova L, Bartikova H, Szotakova B, Lamka J, Varady M and Skalova L. 2013. Biotransformation of albendazole and activities of selected detoxification enzymes in *H. contortus* strains susceptible and resistant to anthelmintics. *Vet. Parasitol.*, 196: 373-381.

Woodgate RG and Besier RB. 2010. Sustainable use of anthelmintics in an integrated parasite management program for sheep nematodes. *Anim. Prod. Sci.*, 50: 440-443.

Chapter 7

Alternative Strategies to Control Trematode Infections in Livestock

A.K. Jayraw, G. Das, V. Agrawal, M. Shakya, G.P. Jatav and N. Jamra*

Department of Veterinary Parasitology,
College of Veterinary Science and Animal Husbandry
NDVSU, Mhow – 453446, Madhya Pradesh
**Department of Veterinary Parasitology,*
College of Veterinary Science and Animal Husbandry,
NDVSU, Jabalpur, Madhya Pradesh

Worldwide, trematodes are responsible for causing highly pathogenic diseases in animals and human beings. The Digenea is one of the largest groups of platyhelminths and infects a wide range of animals including human beings. They affect numerous organs like intestine, lungs, liver, and vascular system of the final host. These trematodes are not only responsible for colossal monetary losses in the livestock industry but are also responsible for decrease in the quality-of-life of human beings (Mas-Coma *et al.*, 2005; Piedrafita *et al.*, 2010; Fürst *et al.*, 2012; Walz *et al.*, 2015 and Qian *et al.*, 2016). Fasciolosis causes substantial monetary losses to the end users like animal owners and landless farmers which is estimated to the tune of US$ 2 billion per year owing to death of infected cattle, liver condemnation and productivity losses due to reduced feed conversion quality. Fasciolosis is widespread in tropical areas which affects 90 per cent of cattle and hence it is considered as the most significant helminth parasite (Mehmood *et al.*, 2017). *Fasciola* infections affect weight gain, milk production, milk solids content and fertility of cattle (Black and Froyd, 1972 and López-Díaz *et al.*, 1998). At present, fasciolosis is considered as an emerging disease in human beings. The World Health Organization has anticipated that 180 million people are at risk of infection and 2.4 million people are infected with fasciolosis in more than 60 countries. Fasciolosis in people is responsible for a decrease in the quality of life. Although paramphistomes (rumen flukes) are generally considered as parasites of less importance in animal health, however, presently, the incidence of amphistomosis has been increased in cattle and sheep. Till date, more than 70 species of paramphistomes have been identified throughout the world.

For control of trematodes, many anthelminthics like triclabendazole, oxyclozanide, rafoxanide and praziquantel are being used. Triclabendazole has been the drug of choice to treat liver fluke infections in livestock for > 20 years, due to its high activity against both adult and juvenile flukes. In addition, it has been used successfully to treat human cases of fasciolosis. Resistance against triclabendazole has been reported for the first time in Australia in mid-1990s. After that, the resistance has been reported from a number of countries throughout the Europe like Ireland, Scotland, Wales, Spain and The Netherlands. The total dependency on a single drug puts the treatment strategies for fasciolosis at risk (Brennan *et al.*, 2007). Ortiz *et al.* (2013) recorded resistance against triclabendazole in *Fasciola hepatica* isolated from dairy cattle of Peru. Therefore, for the control trematode infections, alternative strategies are being developed. Main purpose of the control strategies should be the reduction of transmission rates. Several control methods include the cultural, chemical and biological control.

Control of Snail Intermediate Hosts

Control of snail intermediate hosts is necessary to prevent contamination of the environment by cercariae and metacercariae.

Mechanical Methods

Elimination of breeding places can be achieved by draining of marshy places and by removal of aquatic vegetation mechanically or by using weed killer chemicals like agroxone. Nets and screens should be used to remove the snails from the water bodies. Drainage of water from the water bodies. Snails can be trapped by using palm or coconut tree leaves. Vegetations hanging over the water bodies should be cleared.

Chemical Methods

Chemicals used for snail control are categorized as attractants, contact poisons or repellants. Molluscicides have been used successfully as a short-term control method of snails and can be a cost-effective method; however, this method has not been accepted widely. The main reason for little acceptance of this method is pollution of the environment and killing of non-targeted aquatic organisms. Another reason is rapid recovery of snail population during brief period of favourable conditions, recolonisation takes place which require regular molluscicide application. Molluscicides have mainly been used in dams, as it is a costly affair to use it in the more extensive habitats like rivers. Therefore, snail control by using the molluscicides, in the grazing areas is very difficult owing to the widespread distribution of the snail habitats, very high biotic potential of the snails and the recurrent labour and equipment costs.

Copper Sulphate

It is used @ 10 ppm. For running water copper sulphate bags can be placed at one end of the stream which is effective up to 1.5 km. In ponds, copper sulphate bags can be dragged along the edges. One part of the copper sulphate is mixed with 4 parts of sand and this mixture is spread over the pastures. Copper sulphate @ 22.5 kg/ha of 0.5 per cent solution has been recommended. However, this may be dangerous in areas where chronic copper poisoning used to occur. Copper sulphate kills *Radix luteola, Gyraulus convexiusculus, Indoplanorbis exustus* and *Melanoides tuberculata.*

Copper Pentachlorphenate

It is much more effective as a molluscicide than copper sulphate. When applied @ 11.2 kg/ha in a high-volume spray of 4500 l/ha, it has the advantage of not being inactivated by organic matter. It kills *Indoplanorbis exustus, Radix luteola, Gyraulus convexiusculus* and *Melanoides tuberculata.*

Baylucide

It has the ability to kill *Indoplanorbis exustus, Radix luteola, Gyraulus convexiusculus* and *Melanoides tuberculata.*

Frescon

Tritilomorpholin @ 0.45 kg in 680 litres per hectare can be used as a spray. Two applications in a year are very much useful. It is most effective in small, low-density snail habitats.

Aqualin

It contains acrolein which is effective against snails, their eggs and cercariae.

Sodium Arsenite

Pentile, a 40 per cent commercial solution is used as a spray in the form of a 0.5-1.0 per cent solution. However, it is expensive and poisonous to vegetation.

Metaldehyde

It is used to control land snails and slugs. These baits are often mixed with calcium arsenate or sodium fluosilicate to make the product more effective.

Biological Methods

Several biological agents including some species of algae, bacteria, flies, fungi, nematodes and plants can adversely affect the reproduction or growth of snails. Several competitors, predators and parasites have been used for the control of medically important snails. In the water bodies, snails are infected by leeches, oligochaetes, trematodes, nematodes, fungi and bacteria. Certain species of insects, arachnids, crustaceans, fishes, amphibians, reptiles, birds and mammals prey on the snails.

Plants

Some plants are molluscicides, planting these plants, shrubs along the stream and irrigation channels reduces the snail population. Fruits of *Balanites aegyptiaca, Sapindus emarginatus, Acacia coincinna* (Shikakai), *Caesalpinea corariai* are used to control the snail population. Mahua (*Mahua indica*) seed cake extract is used to kill *Indoplanorbis exustus.* Neem, papaya and eucalyptus leaf extracts have been found effective against *Indoplanorbis exustus* and *Lymnaea luteola.*

Fishes

Rearing of fishes like Gourami and guppy is useful as they swallow the eggs and young snails.

Ducks

Introduction of ducks in the ponds, lakes and paddy fields is useful as they eat snails.

Larvae of flesh fly (*Sarcophaga misera*) acts as a predator for *Indoplanorbis exustus.* Larvae of fire fly thrive on eggs of snails. Larvae and adults of sciomyzid flies, *Sepedon macroplus, Dechaetophora hendeli* and *D. biroi* are efficient killers of snails. The water bug, *Sphaerodemaan nulatum* was found to attach on *Lymnaea accuminata.* Introduction of predatory snails, *Zonitoides nitidus, Oxychilus draparnaudi* and *Physafontalis* were found to control *Lymnaea truncatula.*

Cultural and Husbandry Control

Cultural and husbandry control methods include practices like reducing the stocking rates, rotational grazing and provision of clean grazing. The practical method to prevent amphistomosis, fasciolosis and schistosomosis is to keep the animals away from potentially contaminated water habitats. Although, drainage or fencing-off of wet areas prevents infection of pastures, however, it is a costly affair on grazing land in developed countries and it is very difficult to adopt in developing countries. Complete separation of animals from snail-infested areas is the only practical method in intensive system of farming. Fencing snail-infested waters and supplying cercariae-free water in troughs controlled the *Schistosoma mattheei* infection in cattle on a South African farm. Hence, cultural and husbandry control methods can be applicable in the commercial farming areas.

Improved Drainage

Irrigation projects used to provide the ideal habitat to the snails. Regular clearing of vegetation from drainage channels used to reduce silting and blockages that normally support snail – contaminated herbage. Seepages from irrigation channels also harbour large snail colonies. In low-lying areas, adequate drainage prevents water accumulation. Snails used to multiply for longer duration in wet, low-lying areas. Draining marshy pastures and building dams will be useful to reduce the snail habitats and to increase the grazing area.

Fencing

The snail-infested pastures used to occupy only a small part of animals' grazing area. Fencing off these contaminated areas is a most economic and efficient method for controlling trematode infection, which may prevent a serious outbreaks of trematode infections.

Grazing Management

By adopting the proper grazing management, treatment frequency can be reduced for treatment of trematode infected animals. For that purpose, snail-infested pastures need to be identified. In this case, only those animals should be treated, who are grazing or have grazed the snail-infested pastures.

Managemental Control

Dung of animals should be disposed properly. The wall of manure pit should be made up of concrete and high enough from the ground. The grazing of animals in the contaminated pasture should be restricted. Animals should be dosed near summer and in early rainy season. The silage should be provided to minimize the infection rate in enzootic area.

In future, the alternative methods along with early diagnosis and treatment need to be followed for trematode control. As particularly in case of *Fasciola,* only one drug is available against both the immature and mature *Fasciola.* Hence, its judicious use is warranted owing to the widespread development of the resistance against triclabendzole.

REFERENCES

Black, N.M. and Froyd, G. (1972). The possible influence of liver fluke infestation on milk quality. *Veterinary Record,***90**: 71-72.

Brennan,G.P., Fairweather, I.,Trudgett,A .,Hoey, E., McCoy, M., McConville, M., Meaney, M. Robinson, N., *et al.* (2007). Understanding triclabendazole resistance. *Experimental and Molecular Pathology,* **82**(2): 104-109.

Fürst, T., Keiser, J. and Utzinger J. (2012). Global burden of human food-borne trematodiasis: a systematic review and meta-analysis. *Lancet Infectious Diseases,***12**: 210 - 221.

López-Díaz, M.C., Carro, M.C., Cadórniga, C., Díez-Baños, P. and Mezo, M. (1998). Puberty and serum concentrations of ovarian steroids during prepuberal period in Friesian heifers artificially infected with *Fasciola hepatica*. *Theriogenology*, **50**: 587-593.

Mas-Coma, S., Bargues, M.D. and Valero, M.A. (2005). Fascioliasis and other plant-borne trematode zoonoses. *International Journal of Parasitology*, **35**: 1255-1278.

Mehmood, K., Zhang, H., Sabir, A.J., Abbas, R.Z., Ijaz, M., Durrani, A.Z., *et al.* (2017). A review on epidemiology, global prevalence and economical losses of fasciolosis in ruminants. *Microbial Pathogenesis*,**109**: 253-262.

Ortiz, P., Scarcella,S., Cerna, C., Rosales,C., Cabrera, M., Guzmán, M., Lamenza, P. and Solana, H. (2013). Resistance of *Fasciola hepatica* against Triclabendazole in cattle in Cajamarca (Peru): A clinical trial and an *in vivo* efficacy test in sheep. *Veterinary Parasitology*,195**(1–2)**: 118-121.

Piedrafita, D., Spithill, T.W., Smith, R.E. and Raadsma, H.W. (2010). Improving animal and human health through understanding liver fluke immunology. *Parasite Immunology*, **32**: 572-581.

Qian, M.B., Utzinger, J., Keiser, J. and Zhou, X.N. (2016). Clonorchiasis. *Lancet*. **387**: 800-810.

Walz, Y., Wegmann, M., Dech, S., Raso, G. and Utzinger, J. (2015). Risk profiling of schistosomiasis using remote sensing: approaches, challenges and outlook. *Parasites and Vectors*. **8**: 163.

Chapter 8

Endophytes: Combating Weapon against Microbes and Antheliminitic Resistance

R.K. Sharma and S.K. Jain

Department of Veterinary Pharmacology and Toxicology, College of Veterinary Science and Animal Husbandry, NDVSU, Jabalpur, Madhya Pradesh

Introduction

Helminths are a diverse group of parasitic worms, encompassing nematodes, cestodes and trematodes, and constitute a major health problem for humans and animals in many parts of the world (Kaplan, 2004; Hotez *et al.*, 2008). Although their diseases impact could be reduced dramatically by improved sanitation for humans and pasture control in domestic animals, such methods are not sufficient to eradicate these parasites. In the absence of vaccines, control of these parasites is reliant on chemotherapy to ease symptoms and reduce transmission. The intensive use of drugs in the live-stock industry has led to widespread resistance to all current anthelmintics (Wolstenholme *et al.*, 2004). With few new drugs or vaccines, the fight against parasites could become a losing battle. Understanding the development of drug resistance in parasitic helminths is crucial to prolonging the efficacy of current anthelmintics and developing markers for monitoring drug resistance. It will also be beneficial in the design of new chemotherapeutic agents to overcome or prevent resistance and the identification of new drug targets (Batram *et al.*, 2012). Helminthic diseases are treated with a variety of drugs including macrocyclic lactones, benzimidazoles, imidazothiazoles and praziquantel. In animals, resistance to anthelmintics occurred rapidly after their introduction. There is considerable debate about the definition of resistance, and 'tolerance' is used to describe the stage between success and failure of drug treatment. However, as stated by Coles (2006), resistance occurs when a susceptible population shows any decrease in response to treatment and is complete when the maximum dose of drug that can be tolerated by the host has no effect. Unfortunately, the reduction in response can manifest in different ways, either as a heritable decline in the efficacy of an anthelmintic against a population of parasites that is generally susceptible to that drug or as a decrease in the time a drug treatment exerts its effect, with resistant populations requiring more frequent treatments than previously administered. In an attempt to provide a scientific basis for resistance, resistance has been identified by an increase in the proportion of organisms in a population carrying a gene demonstrated to be linked with resistance (Prichard, 2007). These heritable changes can be either genetic (including mutations, deletions or amplifications of specific genes) or epigenetic (where by methylation of genes or promoter regions of the genes change the gene expression in response to the drug) (Fojo, 2007)

Development of Anthelmintic Resistance

The general consensus is that anthelmintic resistance appears to be a pre-adaptive heritable phenomenon with the gene or genes conferring resistance being present within the parasite population even prior to the drug being used for the first time (Silvestre and Humbert, 2002). Under these circumstances resistance arises as a result of selection through exposure of the worm population to an anthelmintic. When an animal is optimally exposed to an anthelmintic the only worms that should survive are those that carry the genes that confer resistance. For a short period (until the animal becomes re-infected with drug susceptible worms from pasture) the resistant survivors are the only worms laying eggs and in this way the gene pool for resistance is increased.

The indiscriminate use of chemical anthelmintics and the development of resistant strains of parasites for chemical anthelmintics have enforced the search for sustainable alternatives. The herbal anthelmintic approach may be an alternate therapy for the effective control of parasitic infestation and also to combat parasitic resistance against the chemical anthelmintics. The traditional medicines hold a great promise as source of easily available effective anthelmintic agents to the people and animals, particularly in tropical developing countries, including India. The origin of many effective drugs is found in the traditional medicine practices and in view of this, it is important to undertake studies pertaining to screening of the folk fore medicinal plants for their proclaimed biological efficacy. Drug development from plant based compounds could be useful in meeting the demand for newer drugs with minimal side effects.

Endophytes

Endophytes, by definition, is one which resides in the tissues beneath the epidermal cell layers and causes no apparent harm to the host (Stone *et al.*, 2000). They form inconspicuous infections within tissues of healthy plants for all or nearly all their lifecycle (Limsuwan *et al.*, 2009). Studies have shown that, nearly 300,000 plant species that exist on the earth, each individual plant is the host to one or more endophytes, the population of a given endophytic species varies from several to a few hundreds strains (Strobel and Daisy, 2003; Huang *et al.*, 2007). There is a complex relationship between endophytes and their host plants. It is believed that endophytes indirectly benefit plant growth by producing special substances mainly secondary metabolites to prevent the growth or activity of plant pathogens.

Originally, the term endophyte was introduced by De Barry and was assigned to all those microbes that reside inside the living healthy tissues of the plants. Later, this term was expanded as fungi and bacteria including actinomycetes, which spend the whole or at least a part of their life cycle colonizing inter- or intracellularly, inside the healthy living tissue of the host plant, typically causing no apparent symptoms of disease (Verma *et al.*, 2006). Endophytic bacteria living within plant tissues as biotrophic symbionts and these bacteria can be either obligate or facultative. Some endophytic bacteria are able to colonize thousands of different plant species, while some are restricted to plant families. Endophytic bacteria produce a wide range of phytohormones such as auxins, cytokinins and gibberellins. In addition, endophytic bacteria help to enhance the nutrient ability and fix nitrogen for plants (Mahajan *et al.*, 2014).

Along with the production of novel chemicals, many endophytes have shown the capacity for xenobiotic degradation or may act as vectors to introduce degradative traits. The ability of some endophytes to show resistance to heavy metals/antimicrobials and degrade organic compounds probably stems from their exposure to diverse compounds in the plant/soil niche (Ryan *et al.*, 2008).

Classification of Endophytes

Endophytes include a wide variety of microorganisms including fungi, bacteria and viruses. There are two different means of classifying endophytes.

Systemic and Non-systemic

The first method divides endophytes into two categories: systemic (true) and non-systemic (transient). These categories are based on the endophyte's genetics, biology, and mechanism of transmission from host to host. Systemic endophytes are defined as organisms that live within plant tissues for the entirety of its life cycle and participate in a symbiotic relationship without causing disease or harm to the plant at any point. Additionally, systemic endophytes concentrations and diversity do not change in a host with changing environmental conditions. Non-systemic or transient endophytes on the other hand vary in number and diversity within their plant hosts under changing environmental conditions. Non-systemic endophytes have also been shown to become pathogenic to their host plants under stressful or resource limited growing conditions (Heijden *et. al*, 2015).

Biodiversity of Bacterial Endophytes

The endophytic niche offers protection from the environment for those bacteria that can colonize and establish within plants. These bacteria generally colonize the intercellular spaces and they have been isolated from all plant compartments including seeds. Classical studies on the diversity of bacterial endophytes have focused on characterization of isolates obtained from internal tissues following disinfection with sodium hypochlorite or similar agents. Diversity associated with bacterial endophytes exists, not only in the plant species colonized but also in the colonizing bacterial taxa. Plants can be colonized simultaneously by a large variety of endophytic bacteria. The variation in bacteria that has been reported as endophytes spans a significant range of Gram-positive and Gram-negative bacteria and include genera such as *Acidovorax, Acinetobacter Actinomyces, Aeromonas, Afipia, Agrobacterium, Agromonas, Alcaligenes, Alcanivorax, Allorhizobium, Alteromonas, Aminobacter, Aquaspirillum, Arthrobacter, Aureobacterium, Azoarcus, Azo- monas, Azorhizobium, Azotobacter, Azospirillum, Bacillus, Beijerinckia, Blastobacter, Blastomonas, Brachymonas, Bradyrhizobium, Brenneria, Brevundimonas, Burkholderia, Chelatobacter, Chromobacterium, Chryseomonas, Comamonas, Corynebacterium, Delftia, Derxia, Devosia, Enterobacter, Flavimonas, Flavobacterium, Flexibacter, Frankia, Halomonas, Herbaspirillum, Matsuebacter, Mesorhizobium, Moraxella, Nevskia, Nocardia, Ochrobactrum, Pantoea, Pectobacte- rium, Phenylbacterium, Phyllobacterium, Photo- bacterium, Porphyrobacter, Pseudoalteromonas, Pseudomonas, Psychrobacter, Ralstonia, Renibac- terium Rhizobacter, Rhizobium, Rhizomonas, Rhodanobacter, Rhodococcus, Shewanella, Sinorhizobium, Sphingobacterium, Sphingomonas, Spirillum, Stenotrophomonas, Streptomyces, Thauera, Variovorax, Vibrio, Xanthomonas, Xylella, Zoogloea, Zymobacter, Zymomonas,* or members of the group of the pink-pigmented fac- ultatively methylotrophic bacteria, such as *Methylobacterium*. Even though it remains difficult to compare earlier and more recent studies that identify bacteria, certain trends are apparent with predominant bacterial types isolated as endophytes (Lodewyckx *et al.*, 2002).

It should be noted that attempts to evaluate total populations of bacteria in plants may produce varied results, depending on the growth media used for isolation, variations in the growth conditions of the host plant, and the manner in which the plant tissue was used. Molecular approaches for the isolation and characterization of bacterial endophytes and plant-associated bacteria and communities have been reviewed recently by Franks *et al.* (2006). Microbial communities inhabiting stems, roots and tubers of various varieties of plants were analysed by16S rRNA gene-based techniques such as terminal restriction fragment length polymorphism analysis, denaturing gradient gel electrophoresis as well as 16S rRNA gene cloning and sequencing. Generally, colonization by non-pathogenic, endophytic bacteria rarely results in population levels commonly observed for pathogenic bacteria in diseased plant tissue. The number of pathogenic bacteria can range from 1×10^7 CFU/g fresh weight, for example, for *Clavibacter michiganensis* subsp. *sepedonicus* on tomato to $1 \times 10^9 - 1 \times 10^{10}$ CFU/g fresh weight under severe disease pressure, as reported for *Ralstonia solanacearum* on tomato and eggplant (Grimault and Prior, 1994). Contrary to these high concentrations of pathogenic bacteria, common population sizes of introduced endophytic bacteria vary between 1×10^3 and 1×10^5 CFU/g plant tissue for most investigated plant species. Similar to indigenous endophytes, which are usually abundant in the same concentration range as the intro- duced endophytes, the highest bacterial densities are usually observed in the roots and decrease progressively from the stem to the leaves. Independent of the initial inoculum size, endophytic populations tend to approach optimal densities depending on the plant tissue.

Isolation of Endophytic Bacteria

The plant parts were treated with double distilled water for 2-3 minutes and surface sterilized with 0.1 per cent sodium hypochlorite for 5 minutes, 0.01 per cent bavistin for 5 minutes, 0.05 per cent streptomycin for 5 minutes and 70 per cent ethanol for 5 minutes. The plant parts are excised with autoclaved scalpel and forceps in laminar air flow chamber. King's B media or Nutrient agar is used for the isolation of endophytic bacteria (Mahajan *et al.*, 2014). Characterization of bacteria will be done according to its morphology and by Gram's staining. Sun *et al.* (2013) had conducted a study on isolation, characterization and antimicrobial activity of endophytic bacteria from *Polygonum cuspidatum*. The result of the study shows that the endophytic bacteria in *P. cuspidatum* belong to five orders namely Actinomycetales, Bacillales, Rhizobiales, Pseudomonadales and Enterobacteriales. The endophytic bacteria isolated from *P. cuspidatum* shows inhibitory activity against pathogenic fungi and bacteria.

Pal and Paul (2013) had conducted a study on bacterial endophytes of the medicinal herb *Hygrophila spinosa* and their antimicrobial activity. In this study bacterial endophytes were isolated from healthy plant tissues following surface sterilization and plating on nutrient agar, glycerol asparagine agar and tryptic soy agar. They were charactesrized physio-biochemically following standard microbiological and biochemical methods. These endophytes were screened for production of antimicrobial compounds against test strains *Bacillus subtilis, Bacillus cereus, Escherichia coli, Pseudomonas cepacia, Klebsiella pneumonia* and *Staphylococcus aureus* on nutrient agar plates. Eleven phenotypically distinguishable bacterial endophytes were isolated from surface sterilized leaf, stem and root tissues.

Screening of Antimicrobial Natural Products

Crude extracts from the fermentation broth of each endophyte need firstly to be tested through some commonly used methods such as paper disc diffusion method, agar dilution assay, disc diffusion assay and mycelia radial growth. Five of sixty-three endophytic fungi, isolated from rhizomes of a traditional medicinal herb *Paris polyphylla* var. *yunnanensis*, showed strong antibacterial activities against four Gram negative bacteria and two Gram positive bacteria. A plenty of researches have reported that endophytes with no certain compound isolated showed antimicrobial activities and some of which were significant. The efficacy of antimicrobial ingredient is indicated by minimal inhibitory concentration (MIC). Thin layer chromatography (TLC) and bio-autography can be used to track antimicrobial ingredients. A mass of endophyte researches are still in the screening stage and the active ingredient need to be isolated (Yu *et al.*, 2010).

Conclusion

Drug resistance is a threatening problem to livestock industry posing very threats to the future welfare and production of livestock throughout the world. The factors considered most significant have been an excessive frequency of treatments and the administration of an inadequate dose (underdosing) particularly latter is true for developing countries. It may be concluded that sustainable control strategies for helminthosis may require an integrated approach incorporating environmental management, and require a combination drug strategy in order to minimize the pressure for parasite adaptation. Thus a constant urgency to discover novel antibiotics against these microorganisms. Endophytes have proven to be rich sources of novel natural compounds with a wide spectrum of biological activities and a high level of structural diversity. Efficient screening mechanisms are crucial for targeting potential bioactive compound. It is believed that screening for antimicrobial compounds from endophytes is a promising way to overcome the increasing threat of drug resistant strains of pathogens as amtimicrobial or anthelmintics.

Chapter 9

Insecticide Resistance: A Major Problem to Manage Sustainable Growth of Animal Husbandry System

S. Ghosh, Anil Kumar Sharma, Kaushlendra Singh, M. Sankar

Entomology Laboratory, Division of Parasitology, ICAR-Indian Veterinary Research Institute, Izatnagar, Bareilly – 243122, Uttar Pradesh

Introduction

Flies, fleas, lice, mites and ticks are causing severe health and economic consequences in the livestock industry directly by reducing the overall efficiency of animals. Some of these arthropods are also responsible for transmitting pathogens of many fatal diseases of animals (Theileriosis, Babesiosis, anaplasmosis, trypanosmiasis, elrichiosis *etc.*) and human (Crimean-Congo haemorrhagic fever, boreliosis, Rocky Mountain spotted fever, relapsing fever and Colorado tick fever, *etc.*). Use of synthetic insecticides such as organochlorines, organophosphates, carbamates, pyrethroids and macrocyclic lactones is the backbone to control arthropods all over the world. However, frequent and indiscriminate applications fostered not only several environmental and health concerns but also widespread development of resistance to almost all the available chemical based acaricides (Nauen, 2007) and added unwarranted toxic or lethal effects on non-target organisms (Milam *et al.*, 2000). Due to several undesirable and unsustainable features of chemical insecticides, the integrated arthropod management has been considered as only sustainable option.

Definition of Resistance

In 1957, the WHO (1957) defined resistance as "the development of an ability to tolerate toxicants which would prove lethal to the majority of individuals in a normal population of the same species." Later, in 1992, the WHO (1992) defined resistance in arthropods as "an inherited characteristic that imparts an increased tolerance to a pesticide, or group of pesticides, such that the resistant individuals survive a concentration of the compound(s) that would normally be lethal to the species."

Types of Resistance

1. Acquired Resistance

Acquired resistance is defined as "resistance that results from heritable decreases in sensitivity to drugs with the passage of time" (Chapman, 1997, Meyer *et al.*, 2012). Normally, drug resistance is a pre-adaptive phenomenon, in which the resistant allele is present in a population as a rare allele. For example, acquired resistance was induced in *Tetranychus cinnabarinus* against two acaricides. There is a direct relationship between the concentration of the drug and the degree of resistance. A strain controlled by one dose of a drug may show resistance when a lower concentration of the same drug is administered (Mitchell, 1996, Lees *et al.*, 2013). Continued exposure to an acaricide results in the removal of the susceptible members of the population with a concomitant increase in the proportion of the resistant strains, *i.e.*, a process of selection for resistance.

2. Cross-Resistance

Cross-resistance is the sharing of resistance among different acaricides with a similar mode of action. A significant pattern of cross-resistance has been shown among two organophosphates (coumaphos and diazinon) and one carbamate (carbaryl) acaricides in several strains of *Rhipicephalus microplus* (Li *et al.*, 2005, Madder *et al.*, 2011, Perez-Gonzalez *et al.*, 2014). Both carbamates and organophosphates acaricides exert their toxic effects on insects or ticks by inhibiting acetylcholinesterase (AChE), a key enzyme critical to the function of the nervous system of invertebrates (Siegfried and Scharf, 2001, Jensen *et al.*, 2011). Insensitivity of AChE is considered as an important mechanism of resistance against carbamates and organophosphates (Fournier and Mutero, 1994, Dawkar *et al.*, 2013).

3. Multiple Resistance

Multiple resistance is resistance to more than one drugs, even though they have different modes of action. In Mexico, Foil *et al.* (2004) has shown a significant presence of multiple resistance to many classes of acaricides including chlorinated hydrocarbons (DDT), pyrethroids, organophosphates and formamidines (amitraz) in the populations of southern cattle ticks, *R. microplus*.

It was observed that target site mutations were the most common resistance mechanism in the Mexican ticks for these chemicals, but multiple resistance against acaricides with different modes of action also leads one to suspect that resistance may be metabolic (Sammataro *et al.*, 2005, Bielza *et al.*, 2007).

4. Insecticide Resistance in different Arthropods of Veterinary Importance

Mites

Dermanyssus gallinae

First evidence of tolerance of the red poultry mite *Dermanyssus* (*D.*) *gallinae* to synthetic pyrethroids and carbamates was reported from Italy in the 1980s (Genchi *et al.*, 1984). A survey in former Czechoslovakia indicated resistance in *D. gallinae* against synthetic pyrethroids, permethrin, tetramethrin and the organophosphate, trichlorfon on a few farms. Resistance to the banned DDT was, however, widespread (Zeman, 1987). Resistance to synthetic pyrethroids in *D. gallinae* has also been reported in France (Beugnet *et al.*, 1997), Sweden (Nordenfors *et al.*, 2001) and Italy (Marangi *et al.*, 2009).

Psoroptes ovis

Resistance in sheep scab to the organophosphate, propetamphos and the synthetic pyrethroid, flumethrin has been reported in the UK (Synge *et al.*, 1995; Clark *et al.*, 1996; Coles, 1998; Bates, 1998). Populations of *Psoroptes* spp. that showed resistance to flumethrin have also showed cross-resistance to high cis cypermethrin (HCC) (Bates, 1998). In addition, there is evidence of moxidectin resistance in *Psoroptes* mites in the UK (Doherty *et al.*, 2018).

Sarcoptes scabiei

Since the availability of ivermectin formulations for animal use in 1980s, it became the most effective and safe treatment for a broad range of endo- and ectoparasites including *Sarcoptes scabiei* (Campbell, 1989). In fact, ivermectin is included amongst the election drugs to treat scabies not only in humans (Pence and Ueckermann, 2002; Papich, 2016; Chosido and Hay, 2019) but also in domestic and wild mammals. In a case study, Terada *et al.* (2010) reported *S. scabiei* infection was clinically refractory to ivermectin treatment of dogs @ 300 µgDkg bw.

Lice

In the last decades, most of the scientific reports are linked to the development of resistance in the biting louse *Bovicola* (*B.*) *ovis*. The resistance factors (RF) of 26X for synthetic pyrethroid, cypermethrin were calculated (Levot *et al.*, 1995). In 1991, a population of *B. ovis* in New South Wales of Australia was found to have a high RF of 642 to cypermethrin, and cross-resistance also conferred to other synthetic pyrethroids (Levot *et al.*,1995). When these lice populations were challenged by cypermethrin backline treatment (pour-on); however, high level resistance was again selected rapidly (Levot, 2012). Resistance against the more recently introduced insect growth regulators (IGR), the benzoyl urea derivatives such as triflumuron and diflubenzuron was confirmed in lice populations using both moulting inhibition test (James *et al.*, 2008) and louse egg hatch test (Levot and Sales, 2008). In India, the indiscriminate and extensive usage of deltamethrin in Ludhiana district of Punjab state for the control of ectoparasites resulted in the development of resistance in lice, *Haematopinus tuberculatus* population (Singh *et al.*, 2015).

Fleas

There are many reports of *Ctenocephalides felis* resistances from different regions of the world to carbamates, organochlorine, organophosphates, pyrethrins and pyrethroids. Resistance ratios (RR50) were typically less than 20 and reports of cross resistance between carbaryl and organophosphate insecticides were also observed (Coles and Dryden, 2014). Results on resistance studies for the synthetic pyrethroids, permethrin and deltamethrin, however, suggested a level of resistance in all isolates, whilst for tetrachlorvinphos only one field-collected isolate from Australia showed a 21-fold resistance at LD50 compared to the reference strains (Rust *et al.*, 2015). Large-scale monitoring of the imidacloprid resistance status in *Ct. felis* has been carried out in Australia, Germany, France, the UK and the USA. About 770 isolates from dogs and 1516 isolates obtained from cats were collected throughout Australia, the United States and Europe and confirmed sustained susceptibility of *Ct. felis* to imidacloprid, despite its extensive use for almost 20 years (Rust *et al.*, 2011; Kopp *et al.*, 2013).

Flies

Reports of different insecticide resistance in the house fly, *Musca* (*M.*) *domestica* is widespread in different parts of the world. Pyrethroid resistance could be confirmed in the laboratory by topical application of the discriminating dose of 2.5 ng cyhalothrin/fly to 15 isolates selected from different field populations. Four out of 21 field populations showed more than 100-fold resistance at the LD95 of bioresmethrin synergised by piperonyl butoxide. The results of cross-resistance observed between the neonicotinoids thiamethoxam and imidacloprid concluded that their use as replacements for each other should be avoided (Kristensen and Jespersen, 2008). Srinivasan *et al.* (2008) reported the development of tolerance against dichlorvos in *M. domestica* collected from Tamil Nadu state of India.

Mosquitoes and Sand Flies

There are numerous reports from different areas of the world that describe the occurrence of resistance in mosquitos and sandflies against commonly used chemical classes (Alexander and Maroli, 2003; Dhiman and Yadav, 2016; Fawaz *et al.*, 2016; Salim-Abadi *et al.*, 2016). Mosquitoes have developed insecticide resistance both as a direct effect of insecticides targeted on them as well as an indirect exposure to insecticide sprayed on agricultural field (Sharma *et al.*, 2004; Bharati *et al.*, 2016; Bharati and Saha, 2017, 2018; Khan *et al.*, 2020).

Likewise, two Italian sand fly populations (*Phlebotomus* (*P.*) *perniciosus* and *P. papatasi*) were found to be susceptible to 3 different insecticides including permethrin compared to a known susceptible laboratory reference strain, based on bioassay tests according to the WHO standard protocols (Maroli *et al.*, 2002). Compiled information linked to resistance in India, phlebotomine sandflies used to be considered highly susceptible to all insecticides; but indiscriminate use poses a problem of resistance, for example, in Bihar, where spraying with DDT has continued since 1976. Resistance to DDT in *Phlebotomus argentipes*, a proven vector of Kala-azar in India, was reported for the first time in a village of Samastipur district (Mukhopadhyay *et al.*, 1987, 1992). Some reports were also published on tolerance developed against pyrethroid α-Cypermethrin and DDT in *P. argentipes* from India (Dhiman and Yadav, 2016; Dinesh *et al.*, 2014).

Sea Lice (Copepods)

Reduced sensitivity of *Lepeophtheirus salmonis* (the salmon louse) to organophosphates, pyrethroids and emamectin benzoate has been documented (Sevatdal *et al.*, 2005; Espedal *et al.*, 2013; Ljungfeld *et al.*, 2014). Surveillance in Norway also revealed reduced sensitivity of *L. salmonis* to azamethiphos and deltamethrin (Grontvedt *et al.*, 2014).

Ticks

Ticks are considered second to mosquitoes as vectors of animal and human diseases, worldwide. According to FAO (2004), 80 per cent of the world cattle population is exposed to tick infestations which are responsible for severe economic losses both through the direct effects of blood sucking and indirectly as vectors of viral, bacterial and parasitic diseases and also producing toxins resulting in major economic impact on farming communities. Integrated tick management (ITM) is advocated as the most sustainable solution in today's perspective. The ITM strategy includes; monitoring of resistance, restricted use of effective acaricides, use of hosts with natural resistance to ticks, pheromone impregnated decoys for attracting and killing ticks, use of biological control agents, phyto-formulations and vaccines.

Globally, widespread and repeated use of these chemicals without applying proper doses has promoted the establishment of resistant tick populations and polluted the environment and food products (Rodriguez-Vivas *et al.*, 2006; Castro-Janer *et al.*, 2010; Klafke *et al.*, 2017; Vilela *et al.*, 2020). Many of the Mexican tick populations have become resistant to multiple acaricides, way back (Li *et al.*, 2004). The cases of *R. microplus* resistance to organophosphates and pyrethroids (Miller *et al.*, 2005, 2007; Davey *et al.*, 2006; Lovis, 2012) are well documented. In immediate past years, strains resistance to amitraz was also found in *R. microplus* populations from Colombia, Brazil, Mexico and Argentina (Furlong and Diagnóstico de la, 1999; Benavides *et al.*, 2000; Miller, 2002; Rodriguez-Vivas, *et al.*, 2007; Cutullé *et al.*, 2013).) The widespread use of macrocyclic lactones (MLs) for parasite control (endo and ectoparasite) and limited choice of alternative acaricides has caused ivermectin resistance in Mexico (Perez-Cogollo *et al.*, 2010). The first documentation of ivermectin resistance in 10 brown dog tick populations (*R. sanguineus*) has been described in Mexico by Rodriguez-Vivas *et al.* (2017). Resistance to fipronil, a phenylpyrazol (PYZ) compound, was also detected (Castro-Janer *et al.*, 2010).

In India, almost all the cattle populations are suffering from tick infestations which results in tremendous loss of production. Besides its effect on growth and production, tick infestations pose a significant threat to the availability of good quality hides and skin for the leather industry and have been estimated to 20-30 per cent reduction in the cost of leather due to tick bite marks (Biswas, 2003). Among the species of ticks infesting cattle in India, *R. microplus* is the most widely distributed and serves as the major vector of economically important pathogens like *Babesia bigemina* and *Anaplasma marginale* (Ghosh *et al.*, 2007). The epidemiology of tick infestations and their vectorial potential has changed significantly due to changed environmental conditions. In this scenario, the control of tick infestation is considered a major factor for sustainable livestock production worldwide and also to control the tick borne zoonotic diseases.

At present in India, tick control is based on large scale repeated use of synthetic acaricides of major classes. Like other parts of the world, due to the long and repeated use of the chemicals without maintaining proper doses, tick populations have developed resistance to different classes of acaricides in India. During the last decade, acaricide resistance is reported in different parts of India (Kumar *et al.*, 2011, 2021; Sharma *et al.*, 2012; Singh *et al.*, 2013; Nandi *et al.*, 2018; Fular *et al.*, 2020; Upadhaya *et al.*, 2020; Bisht *et al.*, 2021).

Resistance Monitoring Tools

A number of tools have been standardized to monitor and surveillance acaricide resistance. For example;

- ☆ Adult immersion test (AIT)
- ☆ Larval packet test (LPT)
- ☆ Larval immersion test (LIT)
- ☆ Quantification of resistance conferring enzymes by biochemical assays.
- ☆ Identification of point mutation by sequence based typing of targeted gene (s)

Acaricide Resistance Pattern in India

After the establishment of discriminating concentrations (DC) of commonly used acaricides, a number of reports of acaricide resistance in tick populations were published from different states of India (Singh *et al.*, 2010, 2012; Kumar *et al.*, 2011, 2016; Sharma *et al.*, 2012; Shyma *et al.*, 2013; Ahanger *et al.*, 2015; Gaur *et al.*, 2016; Dutta *et al.*, 2017; Chigure *et al.*, 2018; Nandi *et al.*, 2018; Ravindran *et al.*, 2018; Godara *et al.*, 2019; Sagar *et al.*, 2020; Shakya *et al.*, 2020; Upadhaya *et al.*, 2020; Bisht *et al.*, 2021; Fular *et al.*, 2021). But the reports are mainly coming from the states where tick researchers are actively working on the subject.

Against Organophosphates (OPs)

Before the establishment of DC for OP compounds, the first report of resistance in *R. microplus* population against malathion was documented in the Punjab state (Rath *et al.*, 2006). After the establishment of DC, the presence of widespread resistance to diazinon was reported in more than sixty Indian isolates of *R. microplus*, collected from six agro-climatic regions of the country and the highest RF of 26.65 (Kumar *et al.*, 2011) was recorded. Further, loss in the efficacy of diazinon in this tick species collected from Bihar, Haryana and Rajasthan has been reported using both larval and adult stages (Ghosh *et al.*, 2015; Gaur *et al.*, 2016).

Against Synthetic Pyrethroids (SPs)

The use of SP compounds is mostly adopted in most parts of the country without maintaining the dose regime. During the past 10 years, resistance to SP compounds is reported from Uttar Pradesh, Uttarakhand, Bihar, Punjab, Haryana, Jammu and Kashmir, Madhya Pradesh, Rajasthan, Maharashtra, Gujarat, West Bengal, Assam, Kerala and Tamil Nadu (Vatsya and Yadav, 2011; Sharma *et al.*, 2012; Kumar *et al.*, 2013; Khajuria *et al.*, 2014; Singh and Rath, 2014; Ahanger *et al.*, 2015; Gaur *et al.*, 2016; Lenka *et al.*, 2016; Gaur *et al.*, 2017; Dutta *et al.*, 2017; Godara *et al.*, 2019). A remarkable decrease in the potency of deltamethrin is observed in the tick populations in the country.

Against Formamidines

The development of resistance against SP and OP group of acaricides has driven the farmers to rely on the formamidine (amitraz) class of acaricides, which was introduced in the market in the year 1972. Amitraz is under use in different states where SP compounds were not working. The first case of amitraz resistance in India was reported from Gujarat state (Singh *et al.*, 2015a) and subsequently, Kumar *et al.* (2014) reported amitraz resistance at the level from I-III in eleven isolates collected from north India with a maximum RF of 27.3 in Sikar isolates from Rajasthan while Dutta *et al.* (2017) reported a low level of resistance in two tick isolates from four districts of Jammu.

Against Macrocyclic Lactones (MLs)

It was proposed that MLs are systemically active against ticks, and are active against other arthropods and nematodes (Taylor, 2001). The easy availability and applicability of the MLs have resulted in excessive use of this compound without maintaining a proper regimen. The selective pressure due to widespread application of MLs during the past few years has triggered the development of resistance in the tick population and the resistance to ivermectin has been reported from Brazil (Klafke *et al.*, 2006, 2010) and Mexico (Perez-Cogollo *et al.*, 2010). In India resistance against IVM has been reported from Punjab, Uttar Pradesh, Bihar and Madhya Pradesh (Singh *et al.*, 2015; Nandi *et al.*, 2018; Sagar *et al.*, 2019). Recently, the initiation of the development of ivermectin resistance in tick populations has been reported from other states of India (Fular *et al.*, 2020; Bisht *et al.*, 2021; Kumar *et al.*, 2021). Still, MLs are working satisfactorily but there is a need to monitor the situation so that the life span of this effective compound can be extended.

Against Fipronil

This is the most recently introduced acaricide in the market, however, failure of efficacy has also been reported (Castro-Janer *et al.*, 2010; Klafke *et al.*, 2017). Recently, Shakya *et al.* (2020) reported the emergence of fipronil resistance in 11 isolates with RF 1.05- 4.1 out of 25 isolates collected from Haryana, Gujarat, Madhya Pradesh, Assam and Uttarakhand states using larval packet test. But the same isolates were susceptible to fipronil when adults were used in the assay protocol. Bisht *et al.* (2021) reported the susceptibility of all the seven isolates from Uttar Pradesh to fipronil. A significant variation of RF between both tests was found, which raises doubt about the suitability of larva-based assays in the screening of fipronil resistance. Although there is a significant difference in the susceptibility of adults and larvae of the same population to a particular acaricide, the larval stage was used for the convenience of the researchers. There is a need to have an uniform and effective protocol for resistance characterization and concomitantly, research workers and the publication house need to be sensitized suitably so, that the data generation and reporting process is scientifically validated.

Possible Mechanism of Development of Resistance

1. Metabolic Detoxification of Enzymes

Ticks are using a detoxifying enzyme system to break down or sequester a broad spectrum of acaricides due to its wide substrate specificity. Metabolic resistance mediated by detoxifying enzymes such as esterases, glutathione S-transferases (GST) and Cytochrome P450 monooxygenases is reportedly involved in conferring resistance against ticks (Crampton *et al.*, 1999; Jamroz *et al.*, 2000; Enayati *et al.*, 2010; Temeyer *et al.*, 2013).

In India, the work in this area was initiated very late due to the paucity of the suitable reference populations. By comparative quantitative assay Kumar Rinesh *et al.* (2013) reported a 4.35 and 2.92 times more expression of esterases using α- and β-naphthyl acetate as substrate in field resistant population in comparison to the reference susceptible population. A significantly elevated level of α- and β- esterases in field tick isolates was reported from different states resistant to pyrethroids (Singh and Rath, 2014; Ghosh *et al.*, 2015; Chigure *et al.*, 2018). A direct correlation between SP resistance and higher activity of esterases has also been reported by Kumar *et al.* (2016) and Nandi *et al.* (2015).

Besides esterases, the higher activity of monooxygenases has also been associated with resistance development. Enayati *et al.* (2010) and Klafke *et al.* (2017a) reported a significantly higher level of cytochrome P450 activity in the resistant population of *R. bursa* from Iran and pyrethroid resistant Coatzacoalcos Mexican population of *R. microplus*, respectively. Ghosh *et al.* (2015) found 2.28 fold increased activity of monooxygenase in seven tick isolates resistant to deltamethrin, cypermethrin and diazinon collected from different districts of Bihar state, India. A significantly higher GST activity (2 to 5 fold) was reported in resistant *R. microplus* collected from Bihar (Ghosh *et al.*, 2015), Punjab (Nandi *et al.*, 2015), Uttar Pradesh (Chigure *et al.*, 2018; Bisht *et al.*, 2021), Uttarakhand (Fular *et al.*, 2021), Haryana and Gujarat states (Kumar *et al.*, 2021).

2. Target Site Insensitivity

The global research efforts have led to the identification of at least ten mutations (SNPs) in the sodium channel gene (Miller *et al.*, 1999; Morgan *et al.*, 2009; Jonsson *et al.*, 2010; Stone *et al.*, 2014; Klafke *et al.*, 2019). Out of these ten SNPs, five SNPs (T2134A, C190A, G215T, T170C and C2136A) were non-synonymous and their association with resistance has been proved (He *et al.*, 1999; Morgan *et al.*, 2009; Stone *et al.*, 2014; Klafke *et al.*, 2019). None of the Indian isolates has found T2134A mutation across multiple studies (Kumar Rinesh *et al.*, 2013; Ghosh *et al.*, 2015; Kumar *et al.*, 2016; Nagar *et al.*, 2018). Morgan *et al.* (2009) reported cytosine to adenine mutation at position 190 (C190A) in the domain II S4-5 linker of the sodium channel gene of pyrethroids resistance in Parkhurst isolates of *R. microplus* from Australia. Later, this mutation was also detected in pyrethroid resistant *R. microplus* population of Brazil (Mendes *et al.*, 2010; Andreotti *et al.*, 2011; Lovis *et al.*, 2012), Argentina (Lovis *et al.*, 2012), South Africa (van Wyk *et al.*, 2016) and West Africa (Stone *et al.*, 2014; Yessinou *et al.*, 2018).

In India, initially, Kumar Rinesh *et al.* (2013) reported the presence of C190A mutation in the sodium channel gene of the pyrethroid resistant *R. microplus*, collected from four different agroclimatic zones of India. Further, reports were documented in subsequent years while characterizing pyrethroid resistance in ticks collected from other states (Ghosh *et al.*, 2015; Kumar *et al.*, 2016; Ghosh *et al.*, 2017; Nagar *et al.*, 2018; Fular *et al.*, 2018). To date, only C190A point mutation was recorded in pyrethroid resistant Indian *R. microplus* population. We are in the process of genotyping field populations based on C190A mutation.

Studies of acaricide resistant *R. microplus* ticks have shown that esterases, particularly carboxylesterase (CaEs) are associated with resistance. Hernandez *et al.* (2000) detected a higher transcript of carboxylesterase in pyrethroid resistant *R. microplus* population compared to susceptible ticks, suggestive of its role in resistance development. In later studies, this carboxylesterase marker has also been associated with organophosphate resistance in *R. microplus* (Baffi *et al.*, 2007; Faza *et al.*, 2013). However, in extensive studies focusing on multiple isolates collected from different parts of the country, Nagar *et al.* (2016, 2018) did not detect any such mutation at position 1120 in the CaES gene in reference resistant IVRI-IV and IVRI-V strains and in any of the field isolates of *R. microplus.*

Being the target of organophosphates acaricides, AChE are the enzymes of interest to understand the molecular basis of organophosphates resistance. In *R. microplus,* three AChE genes were characterized as AChE1, AChE2 and AChE3 (Baxter and Barker, 1998; Hernandez *et al.*, 1999; Temeyer *et al.*, 2004). In India, the information regarding mutations in any of the AChE genes was scanty, until four amino acid substitutions in AChE2 gene of resistant isolates of *R. microplus* collected from the state of Bihar were identified by Ghosh *et al.* (2015). They suggested that these mutations could probably be associated with organophosphates resistance but the actual contribution of these mutations in the development of insensitive AChE2 could not be ascertained yet. Later, Nagar *et al.* (2016) studied the role of mutations in the AChE2 gene in the development of organophosphates resistance in *R. microplus* and established four amino acid substitutions (viz. V297I, S364T, H412Y and R468K) in the resistant field population and in reference resistant strain of *R. microplus*, as detected earlier by Ghosh *et al.* (2015). Recently, Fular *et al.* (2018) identified 22 SNPs in AChE2 gene in reference multi-acaricide resistant strain (IVRI-V) of *R. microplus* and amino acid substitution was detected in 11SNPs. Although at this stage of research, the presence of various mutations in AChE2 gene of OP resistant Indian isolates of *R. microplus* cannot be correlated conclusively with resistance, however, it provides an insight into one of the possible mechanisms. Jyoti *et al.* (2016a) reported six point mutations and their corresponding amino acid changes in AChE3 gene (I48L, I54V, R86Q, V71A, I77M and S79P). The first three amino acids were previously associated with OP resistance in the Mexican San Roman strain (Temeyer *et al.*, 2007, 2009) and the other three were reported for the first time in India. They hypothesized that these mutations in Indian ticks are possibly associated with OP resistance but not detected in OP resistant strain and field isolates (Nagar *et al.*, 2016). As such, the definite role of these mutations in conferring resistance could not be ascertained.

Amitraz is a triazapentadiene compound and has been used for the management of tick infestations. The use of amitraz became more frequent when pyrethroid resistance problems started to hinder the tick management activities. Several mutations have been detected to date and the development of a single, comprehensive diagnostic test based on DNA sequence variation alone is likely to be difficult (Jonsson *et al.*, 2018). At present, polymorphisms in octopamine-tyramine receptor and βAOR have some potential for molecular diagnosis of amitraz resistance; however, the diversity of mutations suggests that no single polymorphism can be relied on (Rodriguez-Vivas *et al.*, 2018). In India, very few published literature is available demonstrating the role of octopamine/tyramine (OCT/Tyr) receptor gene of *R. microplus* in amitraz resistance (Jyoti *et al.*, 2021).

Management of Acaricide Resistance

The proposed integrated approaches include pasture alternation and/or rotation combined with limited applications of effective chemical acaricides, strategic use of phyto-formulation, housing management, strengthening of dairy cattle management with alternative feeding technologies such as silage and hay to reduce contact between ticks and cattle, immunization against ticks and ticks borne diseases (de la Fuente *et al.*, 2000; Stutzer *et al.*, 2013). Integrated tick management will substantially reduce the over dependence on acaricides and lessen selection pressure on ticks thus will preserve the efficacy of chemicals and reducing the incidence of acaricide resistance (Jongejan and Uilenberg, 2004). Non-chemical natural product based tick management protocol is shown a lot of promise. The indigenous ethno-veterinary and medicinal knowledge of Indian farmers offer a range of herbs for their insecticidal and acaricidal properties. The acaricidal, growth-inhibiting, anti-moulting and repellent activities of many plants and herbs have been scientifically established. Chhabra and Saxena (1998) provided a compilation of plants having acaricidal properties in the Indian subcontinent. The list of active plants has been improved significantly in recent years (Ghosh *et al.*, 2014), and effective phyto-formulations against acaricide resistant tick population has been developed and commercialized. There is a need to develop national level public-private-partnership on natural product development efforts. The researchers in different parts of the country should focus on the actual problems and possible practical solutions. Screening of activity study can be initiated in most of the Parasitology/entomology laboratories but the activity only is not going to give the final product. There are many steps before developing a product and for that, there is a need to bring a multidisciplinary team of researchers involving organic chemists, formulation chemists, entomologists, an expert in thesynthesis of chemicals.

REFERENCES

Castro-Janer, E., Martins, J.R., Mendes, M.C., Namindome, A., Klafke, G.M., Schumaker, T.T.S., 2010. Diagnoses of fipronil resistance in Brazilian cattle ticks *Rhipicephalus (Boophilus) microplus* using in vitro larval bioassays. Vet. Parasitol. 173, 300–306.

Chigure, G.M., Sharma, A.K., Kumar, S., Fular, A., Sagar, S.V., Nagar, G., Upadhaya, D., Saravanan, B.C., Kumar, R., Ghosh, S., 2018. Role of metabolic enzymes in conferring resistance to synthetic pyrethroids, organophosphates, and phenylpyrazole compounds in *Rhipicephalus microplus*. Int. J. Acarol. 44, 28-34.

de la Fuente, J., Rodríguez, M., García-García, J.C., 2000. Immunological control of ticks through vaccination with *Boophilus microplus* gut antigens. Ann. N. Y. Acad. Sci. 916, 617–621.

Dhiman, R.C., Yadav, R.S., 2016. Insecticide resistance in phlebotomine sandflies in Southeast Asia 834 with emphasis on the Indian subcontinent. Infect. Dis. Poverty 5, 106.

Fular, A., Gupta, S., Sharma, A.K., Kumar, S., Upadhaya, D., Shakya, M., Nagar, G., Ghosh, S., 2020. Standardization of tick specific biochemical tools for estimation of esterases, monooxygenases and glutathione S-transferase for characterization of acaricide resistance. Pestic. Biochem. Phys. 164, 130-139.

Jonsson, N.N., Cutullè, C., Corley, S.W., Seddon, J.M., 2010. Identification of a mutation in the para-sodium channel gene of the cattle tick *Rhipicephalus microplus* associated with resistance to flumethrin but not to cypermethrin. Int. J. Parasitol. 40, 1659–1664.

Jyoti, Singh, N.K., Singh, H., Rath, S.S., 2019. Modified larval packet test based detection of amitraz resistance in *Hyalomma anatolicum* Koch (Acari: Ixodidae) from Punjab districts of India. Int. J. Acarol. 45, 391-394.

Klafke, G.M., Miller, R.J., Barreto, R., Guerrero, F.D., Kaufman, P.E. and Pérez de León, A.A., 2017. Mutation in the sodium channel gene corresponds with phenotypic resistance of *Rhipicephalus sanguineus sensu lato* (Acari, Ixodidae) to pyrethroids. J. Med. Entomol. 54, 1639–1642.

Miller, R.J., Davey, R.B., George, J.E., 1999. Characterization of pyrethroid resistance and susceptibility to coumaphos in Mexican *Boophilus microplus* (Acari: Ixodidae). J. Med. Entomol. 36, 533-538.

Morgan, J.A.T., Corley, S.W., Jackson, L.A., Lew-Tabor, A.E., Moolhuijzen, P.M., Jonsson, N.N., 2009. Identification of a mutation in the para sodium channel gene of the cattle tick *Rhipicephalus* (*Boophilus*) *microplus* associated with resistance to synthetic pyrethroid acaricides. Int. J. Parasitol. 39, 775–779.

Nandi, A., Sagar, S.V., Chigure, G., Fular, A., Sharma, A.K., Nagar, G., Kumar, S., Saravanan, B.C., Ghosh, S., 2018. Determination and validation of discriminating concentration of ivermectin against *Rhipicephalus microplus*. Vet. Parasitol. 250, 30–34.

Perez-Cogollo, L.C., Rodriguez-Vivas, R.I., Ramirez-Cruz, G.T., Miller, R.J., 2010. First report of the cattle tick *Rhipicephalus microplus* resistant to ivermectin in Mexico. Vet. Parasitol. 168, 165-169.

Rust, M.K., Vetter, R., Denholm, I., Blagburn, B., Williamson, M.S., Kopp, S., Coleman, G., Hostetler, J., Davis, W., Mencke, N., Rees, R., Foit, S., Böhm, C., Tetzner, K. 2015. Susceptibility of adult cat fleas (Siphonaptera: Pulicidae) to insecticides and status of insecticide resistance mutations at the Rdl and knockdown resistance Loci. Parasitol. Res. 114 (Suppl 1), S7–S18.

Sharma, A.K., Kumar, R., Kumar, S., Nagar, G., Singh, N.K., Rawat, S.S., Dhakad, M.L., Rawat, A.K.S., Ray, D.D., Ghosh S., 2012. Deltamethrin and cypermethrin resistance status of *Rhipicephalus* (*Boophilus*) *microplus* collected from six agro-climatic regions of India. Vet. Parasitol. 188, 337–345.

Sharma, S. N., Saxena, V. K., Lal, S., 2004. Study on susceptibility status in aquatic and adult stages of *Aedes aegypti* and *Ae. albopictus* against insecticides at international airports of south India. J. Commun. Dis. 36(3), 177-181.

Singh NK, Haque M, Singh J, Singh H., 2015. Detection of deltamethrin resistance in buffalo louse *Haematopinus tuberculatus*. Buffalo Bulletin. 34, 209–214.

Singh, R., Das, R. K. and Sharma, S. K., 2001. Resistance of sandflies to DDT in Kala-azar endemic districts of Bihar, India. Bull. World Health Organ. 79, 793–793.

Srinivasan, R., Jambulingam, P., Gunasekaran, K., Boopathidoss, P.S. 2008. Tolerance of house fly, Musca domestica L. (Diptera: Muscidae) to dichlorvos (76 per cent EC) an insecticide used for fly control in the tsunami-hit coastal villages of southern India. Acta Trop. 105(2),187-190.

Upadhaya, D., Kumar, B., Kumar, S., Sharma, A.K., Fular, A., Bisht, N., Srivastava, S., Boruah, R.R., Nagar, G., Shakya, M., Nath, T., 2020. Characterization of acaricide resistance in *Rhipicephalus microplus* populations infesting cattle in northeastern India and assessment of local plant extracts for tick management. Vet. Parasitol. 277, 109011. doi: 10.1016/j.vetpar.2019.109011.

Vilela, V.L.R., Feitosa, T.F., Bezerra, R.A., Klafke, G.M., Riet-Correa, F., 2020. Multiple acaricide-resistant *Rhipicephalus microplus* in the semi-arid region of Paraíba State, Brazil. Ticks Tick Borne Dis. 101413.

Chapter 10

Evaluation of *In vitro* Efficacy of Commonly Used Acaricides by using Bioassay Tools

A. Nandi[1]*, Manisha, A.K. Sharma, S. Kumar, Nisha Bisht, M. Sankar and S. Ghosh*

[1]*Assistant Professor,*
Department of Veterinary Parasitology Faculty of Veterinary Science,
WBUAFS, Kolkata – 37, West Bengal
Entomology laboratory, Parasitology Division,
ICAR- Indian Veterinary Research Institute,
Izatnagar, Bareilly – 243122, Uttar Pradesh

Introduction

Acaricidal resistance is a result of accelerated microevolution. Under selection pressure the fittest survive, multiply and spread. It results from the survival and spread of resistant genotypes that have the capability to endure acaricide selection pressures in the environment. Development of resistance to acaricides is an inevitable consequence of acaricide use for tick control. When the frequency of resistant phenotypes increases to a certain level in field populations, control efficacy with the concerned insecticide becomes economically unacceptable.

Resistance is defined as the capacity acquired by individuals of a parasite population that allows them to survive doses of chemicals which are generally lethal to a normal population (Nari and Hansen, 1999). Cross-resistance (CR) is the mechanism used by resistant insect species to survive the chemically related insecticide exposure, using a generic detoxification pattern (Metcalf 1989). Multiple resistance (MR) is the use of various mechanisms to the action of several classes of chemically unrelated insecticides (Metcalf, 1989).

Synthetic acaricides are the most common tick control approach adopted by the cattle owners in India. These chemicals are available over the counter and are applied on infested animals at frequent intervals. Indiscriminate use with incorrect concentrations of acaricides has probably contributed to the development of large scale acaricide resistance in the ticks (FAO, 2004) as already evident by recently published reports from different parts of the country using Larval Packet Test (LPT) and Adult Immersion Test (AIT). However, these bioassays have been standardized in different laboratories of the world. The following sections describe the protocol for the characterization of resistance through bioassay for monitoring of resistance. The bioassays are conducted as mentioned below:

Discriminating Concentration of Acaricides

The established discriminating concentrations (DCs) of chemical acaricides using adults and larvae of reference susceptible strains of *Rhipicephalus microplus* are to be used for resistance characterization. For a new acaricide DC has to be worked out using reference strain by dose response assay using AIT and LPT and the LC_{50} and LC_{95} values are to be calculated following regression analysis. The DC is determined as 2 X LC_{95} values and the determined DC of some key acaricides is given in Table 10.1.

Table 10.1: Discriminating Concentrations of Chemical Acaricides against IVRI Strain I

Acaricides	*DC (in ppm)*		*LC_{50} value (ppm)*	
	AIT	*LPT*	*AIT*	*LPT*
Deltamethrin	59.2	71.0	13.4	11.8
Cypermethrin	698.2	701.4	138.5	242.4
Fenvalerate	4148.0	4085.8	1204.5	1544.0
Diazinon	1270.4	1273.2	372	499.7
Malathion	9526.4	96.6	2764.2	14.4
Coumaphos	195.6	47.8	33.8	8.6
Amitraz	974.8	895.4	165	-
Fipronil	9.46	9.78	1.68	2.4
Ivermectin	93.5	-	21.68	-

Preparation of Concentrations of Acaricides

Technical grade pure chemical acaricides *i.e.*, deltamethrin, cypermethrin, diazinon, amitraz, malathion *etc.* are to be used to prepare the stock solutions in recommended solvents (table 2). For resistance characterization, different working concentrations of acaricides (*i.e.*, x/2, x, 2x, 3x, 4x, 5x *etc.*,) are to be prepared from stock solution. Here, the 'x' is LC_{95} value of the acaricide against reference strain of *Rhipicephalus microplus*. The discriminating concentration (DC = LC_{95} x 2) of particular acaricide can be prepared as follows:

$$\text{Stock conc. (per cent or ppm)} = \frac{\textit{Desired conc. X desired volume}}{\textit{Purity of the technical grade acaricide}}$$

$$\text{Working conc. (per cent or ppm)} = \frac{\textit{Desired conc. X desired volume}}{\textit{Conc. of the Stock}}$$

NB. 1 per cent = 10,000 ppm= 1 gm/100 ml = 1000mg/100ml = 10mg/ml

Table 10.2: Solvent(s) of the Commonly used Acaricides

Acaricides	*Solvent (Stock) (https: //pubchem.ncbi.nlm.nih.gov)*
Deltamethrin	Acetone (500 g/lit) at 20°C
Cypermethrin	Acetone greater than 450 g/lit; Ethanol 337g/lit at 20°C
Fenvalerate	Acetone >450; methanol>450 g/litat 20 °C
Diazinon	Completelymiscible with common organicsolvents, *e.g.* Alcohols, acetone
Malathion	Ethanol, Benzene
Coumaphos	At 20 °C soluble in acetone (23.82 g/100 mL); muchlesssoluble in denaturedalcohol and xylene (0.9 g/100 mL in each)
Fipronil	Acetone 545.9 g/litat 20 °C
Ivermectin	Absolute ethanol with 2 per cent Tween-20 (Eth-T 20)Stock can be stored at -20°C for five weeks

Bioassay

For the AIT, it is important that the engorged female ticks are healthy and are tested as soon as possible after collection (Within 1-2 days after collection). The size and weight of an engorged female tick will influence its egg laying capacity. If female ticks are below a certain weight the eggs produced are no longer proportional to the weight and ticks below this normal weight should be rejected. Ticks from the field that have **already started to lay eggs (4 to 5 days after collection) are not suitable for testing, damaged and discoloured** ticks should also be rejected. An useful approach is to put the ticks under a source of light (*e.g.* a desk lamp), which will cause healthy ticks to move away.

Collection Time

Because most engorged female ticks drop off the host in the early morning, the engorged female ticks can then be collected from the animals and/or from the ground around them.

1 (a): Adult Immersion Test (AIT) for all the common acaricide [except Ivermectin (MLs)]

Materials Required

Fully engorged females, Petri dishes (6 cm diameter), tissue paper, forceps, Whatman filter paper no. 1, stopwatch, prepared working concentrations of chemical acaricides, cotton cloths, rubber bands, desiccators, weighing machine

Protocol

- ✰ Immediately upon arrival at the laboratory, engorged female ticks should be washed, preferably in distilled water to remove undesired materials or any eggs laid during transport. Those that have started laying eggs should not be used for the AIT.
- ✰ Separate the ticks into batches and maintain the 4 replications having five/ten ticks per replication (n=4x5/4x10).
- ✰ Then immerse the pre-weighed ticks in prepared concentrations of acaricides (*i.e.*, x/2, x, 2x, 3x, 4x, 5x *etc.*,) for 2 minutes and are dried on tissue paper.
- ✰ Soak the treated ticks on tissue paper and transfer to petri dishes.
- ✰ Keep the Petri dishes in desiccators placed in BOD incubator maintained at 28°C and 85±5 per cent RH.
- ✰ Observe the tick mortality regularly up to 14 days post treatment (dpt) when untreated control ticks complete oviposition.
- ✰ Take the egg weight laid by the live ticks per replication to observe inhibition of oviposition.
- ✰ Calculate mean tick weight and mean egg weight of each replication

Determine the reproductive data as follows:

(a) Mortality = engorged females that oviposited were considered as live and females that did not oviposit or with small number of **black eggs (non-viable types) are considered to be dead.**

(b) Egg masses on day 14 post AIT

(c) Reproductive index (RI) = $\dfrac{\text{Egg masses (mg)}}{\text{Engorged female weight (mg)}}$

(d) % Inhibition of oviposition (IO) = $\dfrac{\text{RI control - RI treated}}{\text{RI control}}$ X 100

1 (b): Adult Immersion Test (AIT) for Ivermectin (MLs)

- ✰ Collect the engorged females from animal shed and wash them thoroughly in dist. water.

- ☆ The pre-weighed fully engorged females of *R. microplus* will be immersed in X/4, X/2, X, 2X, 4X *etc.* concentrations.
- ☆ Each concentration will be replicated four times and ten adults were used per replication.
- ☆ The adult ticks are immersed for 30 min in a 15 ml centrifuge tube and gently agitated in a shaker at 25°C.
- ☆ Ticks are removed from the flask, dried, and kept in 5.5 × 1.5 cm plastic petri dishes.
- ☆ Then it kept in desiccators placed in BOD incubator maintained at 28°C and 85 ± 5 per cent RH for 14 days to allow egg laying.
- ☆ The control group of ticks are treated with Solvent (1/100 times of Eth-T 20 stock) and is maintained as above. Following parameters are compared:
  - (a) Mortality = engorged females that oviposited were considered as live and females that did not oviposit or with small number of **black eggs (non-viable types) is considered to be dead.**
  - (b) Egg masses on day 14 post AIT
  - (c) Reproductive index (RI) = $\frac{\text{Egg masses (mg)}}{\text{Engorged female weight (mg)}}$
  - (d) % Inhibition of oviposition (IO) = $\frac{\text{RI control} - \text{RI treated}}{\text{RI control}} \times 100$

An example is as follows:

Technical Ivermectin will be dissolved in Eth-TX or Eth-T20 2 per cent (technical ivermectin does not readily dissolve in water). Technical **Ivermectin** 0.1 g will be dissolved in 10 ml Eth-TX 2 per cent to give 1 per cent Ivermectin and a serial dilution will be again prepared in Eth-TX or Eth-T20 2 per cent. Serial dilution:

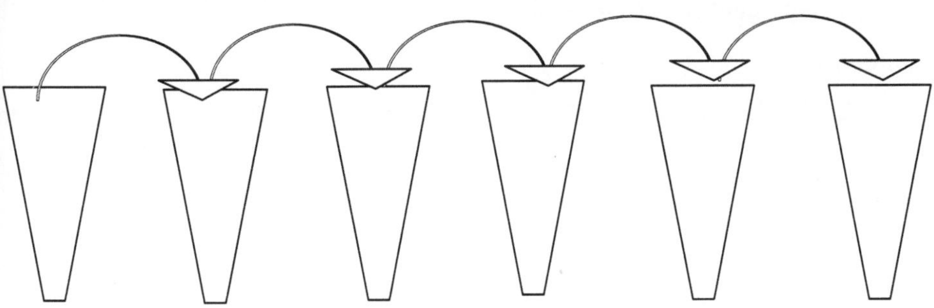

10,000 ppm- ——————————→ 312.5 ppm

In Eth-TX or Eth-T20 2 per cent

Secondary Stock Solutions could be Stored at –20°C for 5 Weeks

Dilution of 1/100 times should be prepared in demineralized water when required. In order toprepare 20 ml solution 0.2 ml of stock solution should be added in 19.8 ml of demineralized water.

$\mathbf{I_1}$ 100 ppm $\mathbf{I_2}$ 50 ppm $\mathbf{I_3}$ 25 ppm $\mathbf{I_4}$ 12.5 ppm $\mathbf{I_5}$ 6.25 ppm $\mathbf{I_6}$ 3.125 ppm

- For preparing all IVM **working solutions,** 1 per cent ethanol and 0.02 per cent Triton X-100 should be used. These are used without MLs as the control solution. **Stability of working solution is 36 hrs. (At temp 4-8°C).**

Table 10.3: Adult Immersion Test (AIT) Laboratory Results Report Sheet for Test of Susceptibility of a Tick Sample against an Acaricide

Isolate name- Date of collection-

Initiation of egg laying: Date of AIT-

Initiation eggs hatching:

	Engorged Female Tick		*Egg Laying (14dpt)*			*Efficacy*		
Conc. of Acaricide	*No. (10 in each)*	*Weight*	*Dead*	*Complete/ Partial (C/P)*	*Weight (g)*	*Mort. per cent*	*RI*	*Hatchability per cent*
10 ppm	R_1	1070	8	P	78	80		90
	R_2	1305	7	P	67	70		90
	R_3	1320	8	P	47	80		90
	R_4	1332	8	P	68	80		80

2. Larval Packet Test (LPT)

Materials Required

Whatman filter paper No.1, scissors, cello tape, pipette, prepared conc. of products, 15 days old larvae, brush.

Procedure

- The LPT is conducted as described earlier (FAO 1971) with minor modifications.
- Prepare the packets in parallelogram shape (approx. 5.5 cm x 5 cm) from Whatman filter paper No.1 **(Fig. 1).**
- Impregnate the packets with 500-600 µl of working solution of acaricide with the help of pipette.
- Use minimum three replication of each concentration.
- Dry the impregnated packets for at least 30 min in incubator at 37 °C.

- ☆ After drying, fold the packets in half and seal on one side with adhesive tapes forming an open-ended packet.
- ☆ Insert approx. 100 larvae (10-14 days old) in the packets with the help of brush from one open side.
- ☆ Now, seal the side of the packet and place in BOD incubator.
- ☆ After 24 h, open the packets under light exposure on white paper encircled with water to prohibit fast movement of larvae.
- ☆ Count the dead and live larvae with the help of brush.
- ☆ The recommended mortality criterion is the inability of tick larvae to walk. Only those larvae capable of walking are considered to be alive.
- ☆ The percentage larval mortality is calculated accordingly.

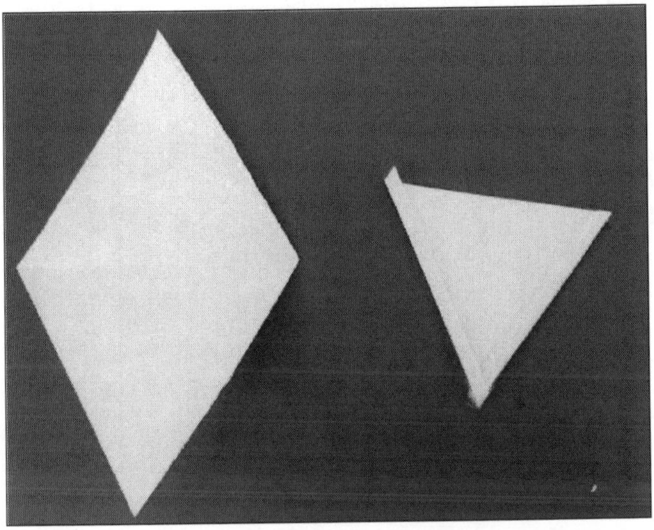

Figure 10.1: Larval Packets (Opened and sealed).

Table 10.3: Larval Packet Test (LPT) Laboratory Results Report Sheet for Test of Susceptibility of a Tick Sample against an Acaricide

Isolate name- Date of LPT-

Date of collection- Acaricide-

Conc. of Acaricide	*Replicate*	*Live*	*Dead*	*Mortality per cent*
50 ppm	R_1	120	0	
	R_2	125	0	
	R_3	100	10	
	R_4	100	5	

REFERENCES

Abbott W S. 1987.A method of computing the effectiveness of an insecticide. *Journal of American Mosquito Control Association* **3**: 302-303.

Kumar S, Paul S, Sharma A K, Kumar R, Tewari S S, Chaudhuri P, Ray DD, Rawat A K and Ghosh S. 2011. Diazinon resistant status in *Rhipicephalus (Boophilus) microplus* collected from different agro-climatic regions of India. *Veterinary Parasitology* **181**: 274-281.

Sharma A K, Kumar R, Kumar S, Nagar G, Singh N K, Rawat S S, Dhakad M L, Rawat A K S, Ray D D and Ghosh S. 2012. Deltamethrin and cypermethrin resistance status of *Rhipicephalus* (*Boophilus*) *microplus* collected from six agro-climatic regions of India. *Veterinary Parasitology* **188**: 337-45.

Drummond R O, Crust S F, Trevino J L, Gladney W J and Graham O H. 1973. *Boophilus annulatus* and *Boophilus microplus:* laboratory tests of insecticides. *Journal of Economic Entomology* **66**: 130–133.

FAO 2004. Guidelinesresistance management and integrated parasite control in ruminants. *Module 1: Ticks: acaricide resistance: diagnosis, management and prevention.* pp. 1 – 53.

Nandi A, Sagar SV, Chigure G, Fular A, Sharma AK, Nagar G, Kumar S, Saravanan BC, Ghosh S. Determination and validation of discriminating concentration of ivermectin against *Rhipicephalus microplus*. *Veterinary parasitology*. 2018 Jan 30; 250: 30-4.

Chapter 11

Demonstration of Metabolic Detoxification Mechanism of Resistance through Biochemical Assay

A. Fular, N. Bisht, D. Upadhaya and A. Nandi

Entomology laboratory, Parasitology Division,
ICAR- Indian Veterinary Research Institute,
Izatnagar, Bareilly – 243122, Uttar Prdaesh

Introduction

The targeted enzyme groups are:

- ☆ Esterases
- ☆ Monooxygenases (Cytochrome P_{450})
- ☆ Glutathione S-transferases

Materials Required for Esterase Assay

Biological sample in multiples of 40 counted larvae were packed in eppendorf tube and stored at -40°C/-80°C.

Equipments/Glass Wares/Plastic Wares

- ☆ Spectrophotometer
- ☆ Refrigerator (-40°C/-80°C)
- ☆ Refrigerated centrifuge
- ☆ pH meter
- ☆ Microtitre plate

- ✰ Prechilled mortar and pestle
- ✰ Beakers and Bottles
- ✰ Micropipettes of variable range

Preparation of Naphthol Standard Curve for Esterase Assay

The product of the reactions with α-Naphthyl acetate and β-Naphthyl acetate are α- and β- Naphthol respectively. Standard curve should be set for the commercially available α and β- Naphthol separately for different range of concentrations (*i.e.* 5 nmoles, 10 nmoles, 15 nmoles and so on) in 220 µl 0.02 M phosphate buffer pH 7.2 with 50 µl of fast blue solution. Measure the absorbance at 570 nm in microplate reader. The data is subjected to linear regression analysis and thus a standard curve is prepared.

Preparation of Monooxygenase Standard Curve

The stock solution of 0.01 mg/ml or 10 µg/ml of cytochrome C is prepared in 0.625M potassium phosphate buffer. In each well, add 20µl cytochrome C, 200 µl of 3,3′,5,5′-tetramethylbenzidine (TMBZ) and 25 µl of 3 per cent H_2O_2. Incubate the plates for 5 min in dark and measure the absorbance at 650 nm. The data is subjected to linear regression analysis and thus a standard curve is prepared.

Preparation of Protein Standard Curve

The protein standard curve is drawn with serially diluted stock solution of standard BSA (2mg/ml; Sigma Aldrich). 10 µl of BSA is added to 200 µl of 1x solution of Bradford reagent (Sigma Aldrich) in each well. The OD is recorded after an incubation of 15 min dark at room temperature at 595 nm in spectrophotometer. The data is subjected to linear regression analysis and thus a standard curve is prepared.

Sample Preparation

- ✰ Homogenize the pre counted 40 deep-frozen larvae for esterase and GST assay using pre chilled mortar pestle.
- ✰ Add150 µl of homogenization buffer.
- ✰ In case of monooxygenase, 80 larvae are used.
- ✰ Run the tick homogenate at 13000 rpm in a refrigerated centrifuge at 4 °C for 15 min.
- ✰ Use the resulting supernatant as enzyme source.
- ✰ The supernatant can also be stored at -40° C or -80°C until used.

Esterase Assay Procedure

Principle

In this method, α-naphthyl and β-naphthyl ester substrates are hydrolyzed by enzymatic action to alpha-naphthol and β-naphthol which couples to fast Blue (a diazonium salt) forming a diazo dye complex. This diazo dye complex is measured by spectrophotometer.

Procedure

[Habig *et al.*, 1974, Hemingway and Brogdon, 1998, Ghosh *et al.*, 2017]

- ☆ Add 20 µl of tick homogenate in adjacent wells in a 96 microtitre plate.
- ☆ Add 20 µl of homogenization buffer in control well.
- ☆ Add 200 µl of working solution of α-naphthyl and β-naphthyl acetate.
- ☆ Incubate the mixtures at room temperature for 15 minutes.
- ☆ Add 50 µl of fast blue solution to each well.
- ☆ Incubated at room temperature for 5 minutes. (Fast blue stain the naphthol produced and SDS stops the reaction)
- ☆ Measure the absorbance at 570 nm in a spectrophotometer.

Monooxygenase Assay Procedure

Principle

The cytochrome P_{450} enzyme also known as monooxygenase. The assay described here does not measure the monoxygenation activity of cytochrome P_{450} enzyme over a substrate, directly, instead it quantifies the total amount of heme content of the larval homogenate and this enables an indirect estimate of the enzyme activity. Hence, the higher the heme content higher should be the enzyme activity.

Procedure

[Brogden *et al.*, 1997, Fular *et al.*, 2018, Upadhaya *et al.*, 2019]

- ☆ Add 20 µl of tick homogenate in a 96 microtitre plate.
- ☆ Add 20 µl of homogenization buffer in control well.
- ☆ Add 80 µl of 0.625 M potassium phosphate buffer (pH 7.2) to each well.
- ☆ Add 200 µl of TMBZ solution to each well.
- ☆ Add 25 µl of 3 per cent hydrogen peroxide.
- ☆ Incubate the plates at 5 min in dark.
- ☆ Measure the absorbance at 650 nm.

The Glutathione-S Transferase Assay Procedure

Principle

GST catalyzes the conjugation of L-glutathione to CDNB through the thiol group of the glutathione.

$$GSH + CDNB \xrightarrow{GST} \text{GS-DNB Conjugate} + HCl$$

The reaction product, GS-DNB Conjugate, absorbs at 340 nm. The rate of increase in the absorption is directly proportional to the GST activity in the sample.

Procedure

[Habig *et al.*, 1974, Fular *et al.*, 2018, Upadhaya *et al.*, 2019]

The reaction mixture in each well of the 96 well microtitre plate is prepared as follows:

- ☆ Add 10 µl of tick homogenate in a 96 microtitre plate.
- ☆ Add 20 µl of homogenization buffer in control well.
- ☆ Add 200 µl of working solution in each well as well as in control wells.
- ☆ Incubate the plate for 200 minutes in dark.
- ☆ Measure the absorbance at 340 nm.

Protein Assay

Principle

The principle of this assay is that the binding of protein molecules to Coomassie dye under acidic conditions results in a color change from brown to blue. This method actually measures the presence of the basic amino acid residues, arginine, lysine and histidine, which contributes to formation of the protein-dye complex.

Procedure

- ☆ Add 10 µl of tick homogenate in a 96 wells microtitre plate.
- ☆ Add 10 µl of homogenization buffer in control well.
- ☆ Add 200 µl of Bradford solution in each well as well as in control wells.
- ☆ Incubate the plates for 15 minutes in dark.
- ☆ Measure the absorbance at 595 nm.

Troubleshooting

- ☆ The substrate used should be from Sigma Aldrich

- ☆ If there is no colour formation then the purity of chemicals might be tossed.
- ☆ The homogenization buffer prepared for the homogenization should be checked with Bradford reagent for reactivity before the start of all the biochemical assays. If found reactive, the homogenization buffer components need to be changed.
- ☆ Age of larvae is important.
- ☆ All the working solutions/reagents other than the buffers should be freshly prepared by proper vortexing.
- ☆ The working solutions such as alpha naphthyl acetate, beta naphthyl acetate, TMBZ solutions and CDNB solutions should be prepared in amber colored bottles.
- ☆ The Bradford reagent should also be taken in amber colored vial for protein determination.
- ☆ The reaction should be established in dark and the ELISA plates when incubated should also be kept in dark.

A. Preparation of Solutions Require for Esterase Assay

0.2 M monobasic sodium phosphate buffer

Monobasic sodium phosphate (dihydrate)	6.24gm
Distilled water up to	200ml

0.2 M dibasic sodium phosphate buffer

Dibasic sodium phosphate	5.68gm
Distilled water up to	200ml

0.1 M sodium phosphate buffer (pH 7.0)

0.2 M monobasic sodium phosphate	117ml
0.2 M dibasic sodium phosphate	183ml
Distilled water	300ml

Adjust pH to 7.0 and keep at 4°C

0.02 M sodium phosphate buffer (pH 7.2)

0.2 M monobasic sodium phosphate-	16.8ml
0.2 M dibasic sodium phosphate-	43.2ml
Distilled water	540ml

Adjust pH to 7.2 and keep at 4°C

30 mM α- Naphthyl acetate solution

α- Naphthyl acetate	27.93mg
Acetone	5 ml

Stored in a tight stoppered bottle at 4°C.

30 mM β-Naphthyl acetate solution

β- Naphthyl acetate	27.93mg
Acetone	5 ml

Stored in a tight stoppered bottle at 4°C

Working solution of α-Naphthyl acetate solution

30mM α- Naphthyl acetate solution	100µl
0.02 M sodium phosphate buffer (pH 7.2)	9900µl

Working solution of β-Naphthyl acetate solution

30mM β- Naphthyl acetate solution	100µl
0.02 M sodium phosphate buffer (pH 7.2)	9900µl

Working solution should be made freshly and used within 1 hour of preparation

5 per cent SDS solution

SDS	2.5gm
0.1 M sodium phosphate buffer (pH 7)	50 ml

Fast blue solution

Fast blue salt	15 mg
Distilled water	1.50ml
5 per cent SDS solution	3.50ml

B. Reagents for Glutathione-S-transferase Assay

0.1 M Potassium Phosphate buffer (pH 6.5)

0.2 M Monobasic potassium phosphate	202.5ml
0.2 M Dibasic potassium phosphate	94.5ml
Distilled water up to	1L

Adjust pH to 6.5 and keep at 40C

10 mM Glutathione

Reduced Glutathione	0.0081g
0.1 M Potassium Phosphate buffer (pH 6.5)	2.5 ml

Keep in ice and use within two hrs, prepare freshly for each assay

63 mM chlorodinitrobenzene (CDNB)

Chlorodinitrobenzene	0.013g
Methanol	1000µl

Keep in ice and use within two hrs, prepare freshly for each assay

Working solution

63 mM Chlorodinitrobenzene	**125µl**
10 mM Glutathione	2500µl

Keep in ice and use within two hrs, prepare freshly for each assay.

C. Reagents for Monooxygenase Assay

0.25 M Sodium acetate buffer (pH 5.0)

Sodium acetate anhydrous	8.2gm
Distilled water up to	400ml

Adjust the pH with glacial acetic acid and store at room temperature.

1M Monobasic potassium phosphate buffer

Monobasic Potassium Phosphate	54.4gm
Distilled water up to	400ml

Autoclaved and stored at 4°C

1 M Dibasic potassium phosphate buffer

Dibasic Potassium phosphate	69.68gm
Distilled water up to	400ml

Autoclaved and stored at 4°C

0.625 M Potassium phosphate buffer (pH 7.2)

1M Monobasic potassium phosphate buffer	28.3ml
1M Dibasic potassium phosphate buffer	71.7ml

Autoclaved and stored at 4°C

Tetramethyl Benzidine solution (TMBZ)

Tetramethyl Benzidine	20mg
Methanol	10ml

Store at 4°C

Working Solution

TMBZ solution	5ml
0.25M Sodium acetate buffer	15ml

The solution should be made fresh.

3 per cent Hydrogen Peroxide

H_2O_2	3ml
Distilled water	97ml

Store at 4°C

Homogenization buffer (100ml)

0.1M Potassium Phosphate buffer (pH=6.5)	100 ml
Sucrose	20 gm
EDTA	37.22 mg

Data Analysis in MS Excel Sheet

Esterase

α- naphthol: y= 0.032x-0.033

β- naphthol: y=0.007x-0.005

1. Homogenate OD= A
2. Control OD= B
3. Corrected OD= A-B= D
4. m α- naphthol = 0.032=, m for β- naphthol = 0.007
5. c= 0.033= α- naphthol, c= 0.005= β- naphthol
6. x= (D+0.033)/0.032= α- naphthol, x= (D+0.005)/0.007= β- naphthol
7. Incubation Period= 15 min
8. x/15= F
9. Protein value= G
10. F/G= H
11. Average of H= enzyme level
12. STDV
13. SE= STDV/√N where N= number of replicates

Each numbers represent cell of excel sheet.

Monooxygenase

Y = 5.671x+0.014

1. Homogenate OD= A
2. Control OD= B
3. Corrected OD= A-B= D
4. m= 5.671
5. c=0.014
6. X= (D-0.014)/5.671
7. Protein value= G
8. GX2= I
9. X/I= K
10. Average of K= enzyme level
11. STDV
12. SE= STDV/√N where N= number of replicates

Glutathione S-Transferase

The concentration of GST was calculated by Lambert-Beer's law;

$$\mathbf{A = \varepsilon CL}$$

where,

A: Absorbance at 340 nm after 15 minutes

ε: Extinction coefficient of product (3-(2-chloro-4-nitrophenyl)-glutathione) = 4.39 mM-1

L: Path length, which in this case was 6 mm.

C: Concentration

For calculating the specific activity of GST,

GST (mM/mg/min) = Optical Density **X** 1000/4.39 mM-1 **X** 6 mm **X** total protein in 10 µl homogenate **X** 20 min.

1. Homogenate OD= A
2. Control OD= B
3. Corrected OD= A-B= D
4. Protein value= G
5. Factor, H= 1.89254
6. (D/G)*H= K
7. Average of K= enzyme level
8. STDV
9. SE= STDV/√N where N= number of replicates

Protein

$Y = 0.0023x+0.2736$

(y=mx+c depends on the Bradford reagent)

1. Homogenate OD= A
2. Control OD= B
3. Corrected OD= A-B= D
4. m= 0.0023
5. c= 0.2736
6. x= (D-0.2736)/0.0023= Required protein value

Chapter 12

Molecular Detection of Acaricide Resistance in Ticks

Rinesh Kumar

Department of Veterinary Parasitology,
College of Veterinary Science and Animal Husbandry
NDVSU, Rewa – 486550, Madhya Pradesh

Introduction

Infestation of cattle with the one host tick, *Rhipicephalus microplus* (*R. microplus*) has been reported from most of the tropical and subtropical countries and it is ranked as the most economically important ectoparasite of the cattle in the world (Angus 1996; Solorio *et al.*, 1999). Its success and impact as an invasive species can be attributed to several factors, like high adaptability as it can displace endemic species (Adakal *et al.*, 2013; George *et al.*, 2004; Lynen *et al.*, 2007; Madder *et al.*, 2011; Nyangiwe *et al.*, 2013; Tonnensen *et al.*, 2004); vector competence for several pathogenic species (*Anaplasma*, *Borrelia* and *Babesia spp.*) (de la Fuente *et al.*, 2007; Jongejan and Uilenberg 2004); voracious blood feeder (Ghosh *et al.*, 2006); as well as rapid development of resistance to major chemical classes of acaricides due to its short and single host life cycle (Martins and Furlong 2001; Li *et al.*, 2005; Li *et al.*, 2007; Castro-Janer *et al.*, 2010; Mendes *et al.*, 2011; Rodriguez-Vivas *et al.*, 2011; Rodríguez-Vivas *et al.*, 2014). Despite efforts to develop vaccines or other non-chemical based methods to control ticks, the use of chemical acaricides is the predominant approach implemented in the field therefore, acaricides remain to be the mainstay of tick control programmes in the near future (Ghosh *et al.*, 2007). For optimum and strategic use of acaricides, to slow down the process of development of resistance in ticks and to obtain knowledge of the distribution pattern of acaricide resistance, there is a need to monitor acaricide resistance in the field. To do so, the Food and Agriculture Organisation (FAO) currently recommends and provides standardised protocols for two bioassays to evaluate tick resistance (2004), the Larval Packet Test (LPT), originally described by Stone and Haydock (1962), and the Adult Immersion Test (AIT), originally developed by Drummond *et al.* (1973).In 2004, White *et al.*, developed an additional test; the Larval Immersion Microassay (LIM) while the Larval Tarsal Test was introduced a few years back (Lovis *et al.*, 2011). The increased length of time by which results from a bioassay are obtained, the need for live tick specimens and the inability to detect the genotype status of resistant individuals, negatively influences the effectiveness of these techniques (Sungirai *et al.*, 2018). Today the major emphasis in research on resistance lies on to divulge the underlying molecular mechanisms and to use this knowledge to control the development and expansion of resistant populations (Leeuwen *et al.*, 2010). In comparison to bioassays, molecular assays have the advantage to provide results within a day, to require very few ticks and to provide confirmatory information about resistance mechanisms. The success of molecular assays depends on the availability of precise molecular markers, which are identified and validated through different molecular tools in the targeted genes. The study of single nucleotide polymorphism (SNP) potentially associated to the acaricide resistance phenomenon is one of the most popular approaches in trying to find molecular markers for acaricide resistance monitoring/diagnostic purposes (Guerrero *et al.*, 2001; Morgan *et al.*, 2009; Rosario-Cruz *et al.*, 2009; Hernandez *et al.*, 2002; Baron *et al.*, 2015). Diverse mutations have been identified in the voltage-gated sodium channel gene in *R. microplus*, which result in insensitivity to pyrethroids (Miller *et al.*, 1999; He *et al.*, 1999; Jonsson *et al.*, 2010; Morgan *et al.*, 2009; Stone *et al.*, 2014). An esterase in a pyrethroid resistant Mexican *R. microplus* strain was isolated and Hernandez *et al.* (2000) found a mutation in the encoding gene, the same mutation was found in organophosphate resistant strains by Baffi *et al.* (2007). Mutations in genes encoding carboxylesterases will increase esterase hydrolytic activity on an acaricide (Jamroz *et al.*, 2000). Chen *et al.* (2007) identified two mutations in a putative octopamine receptor gene and similarly, Corley *et al.* (2013) identified a novel non-synonymous nucleotide substitution in the β-adrenergic octopamine receptor gene of *R. microplus* that will result in target site insensitivity to amitraz resistance. Identification of different SNPs in the acaricide resistant associated gene of *R. microplus* has enabled the researchers to develop the molecular markers (Guerrero *et al.*, 2001; Morgan *et al.*, 2009; Hernandez *et al.*, 2002; Baron *et al.*, 2015) for detection and monitoring of pyrethroid, organophosphate and amitraz resistance. Increasingly, it is possible to describe the genotypic resistance profile of a tick or a population of ticks as molecular markers for resistance against several acaricides becomes available, which can detect the presence of resistance-associated genes in a tick population before it reaches high frequency.

With the availability and affordability of molecular tools, these DNA-based monitoring assays could assist the management of resistance in a very effective way. The purpose of this review is to summarize the gene mutations or SNPs discovered so far, in the targeted acaricide resistance genes of the *R. microplus*. The collection of different SNPs or mutations, which are clearly associated with acaricide resistance or likely to be associated with acaricide resistance, will help us in rapid resistance detection and monitoring.

Mechanisms of Resistance in *R. microplus*

R. microplus ticks have acquired the ability to evade the toxic effects of chemical acaricides by developing different resistance mechanisms, which are generally classified into three main categories: target site insensitivity, increased metabolic detoxification, and reduced cuticular penetration (Guerrero *et al.*, 2012). The cuticle surrounding the tick, which reduces acaricide access to the internal environment of the tick body, confers penetration resistance. Penetration resistance in ticks could arise through alterations in the ability of an acaricide to penetrate or otherwise enter an individual that is treated with acaricide. However, further investigations into this type of resistance in *R. microplus* have not been reported since 1983 (Schnitzerling *et al.*, 1983). Target-site and metabolic resistance are common in *R. microplus* and have been widely studied for some classes of compounds, such as the pyrethroids. Target site resistance occurs when a single nucleotide substitution in the gene coding for the target molecule of an acaricide results in an amino acid change that confers a lower susceptibility to the acaricidal compound (Guerrero *et al.*, 2012). Lastly, metabolic resistance to acaricide treatment involves the increased ability to detoxify or sequester the acaricide. Metabolic resistance mediated by detoxifying enzymes such as esterases, glutathione-S-transferases (GST) and Cytochrome P450 monoxygenases have also been established in the *R. microplus* (Crampton *et al.*, 1999; Jamroz *et al.*, 2000; Baffi *et al.*, 2005; Chevillon *et al.*, 2007; Cossio-Bayuger *et al.*, 2008; Guerrero *et al.*, 2012). The metabolic enzyme system produces resistance by two ways. They got physically changed (an alteration in the catalytic center activity of enzymes which increases the rate at which the enzyme unit metabolize the acaricides) or overproduced (the elevated activity of enzymes, leading to increased metabolism and sequestration) (Hemingway 2004). Chemicals known as synergists are often used to identify the type of enzymes involved in metabolic resistance. Piperonyl butoxide (PBO), triphenyl phosphate (TPP) and diethylmaleate (DEM) are the three most commonly used synergists and are considered to be specific inhibitors for cytochrome P450s, esterases, and glutathione S-transferases, respectively (Guerrero *et al.*, 2012). All of the aforementioned mechanisms have been shown to play a vital role in tick resistance to chemical acaricides.

Monitoring/Diagnosis of Resistance by Molecular Tools

Today, the ability of molecular tools to rapidly detect resistance SNPs and divulge the underlying molecular mechanisms in field populations of *R. microplus* have helped immensely in directing the effort of tick eradication and/or control programs. The sensitivity of these molecular assay is such that the early stages of the spread of resistance genes can be detected quickly and control measures adopted, when available, to slow the spread of these genes and lengthen the period of time which a particular acaricide is efficacious against *R. microplus*.

Various molecular techniques such as target gene amplification, allele-specific PCR, sequencing techniques with DNA, transcriptomic analysis with RNA and probe-based quantitative PCR assays have been developed for detecting acaricide resistance in ticks have helped in rapid detection of resistance and have greatly improved acaricide resistance management. (Guerrero *et al.*, 2001; Hernandez *et al.*, 2002; Chen *et al.*, 2007; Rodriguez-Vivas *et al.*, 2011; Lovis *et al.*, 2012; Sungirai *et al.*, 2018). These molecular-based assays are sensitive and rapid alternatives to bioassays for determining the status of acaricide resistance within a population to enable rational selection of appropriate treatments for parasite control (Jonsson *et al.*, 2010).

Resistance Mechanism for Pyrethroid Resistance

Synthetic pyrethroids (SPs) were introduced in the mid to late 1970s and have been widely used as very effective insecticides and acaricides. They are not very toxic to mammals and are highly biodegradable. *R. microplus* is a major ectoparasite of cattle in tropical and subtropical climates worldwide, it has already developed resistance to several acaricides, and resistance to SP is particularly common in this species. Synthetic pyrethroids resistance has been reported, where the species *R. microplus* is endemic such as in Asia, Africa, North America and South America (Kunz and Kemp, 1994; Jonsson *et al.*, 2000; Rodriguez-Vivas *et al.*, 2006a, Rodriguez-Vivas *et al.*, 2006b; Lovis *et al.*, 2012; Ghosh *et al.*, 2015; Kumar *et al.*, 2013; Bandara and Karunaratne 2017; Yessinoua *et al.*, 2018).

Mutation in Sodium Channel Gene

The first markers of resistance were developed for SPs. He *et al.* (1999) for the first time identified a novel nucleotide substitution of an adenosine (A) for thymidine (T) at position 2134 (T2134A) in a highly conserved domain IIIS6 transmembrane segment of the sodium channel gene (GenBank Accession No. AF134216), resulting in the replacement of a phenylalanine by an isoleucine (F712I) in San Felipe and Corrales strains of *R. microplus* from Mexico that was extremely resistant to pyrethroids. This was followed by the discovery of two new SNPs (C190A, G215T) in domain II S4-5 linker of the sodium channel gene in *R. microplus* (Morgan *et al.*, 2009; Jonsson *et al.*, 2010). Using tick samples from the US and Mexico, Stone *et al.* (2014) confirmed the presence of mutations not only in domain III (T2134A), but also in domain II (C190A) of the para-sodium channel gene associated with SP resistance. Additionally, the authors discovered a putative super-kdr SNP in domain II (T170C) that was previously detected in the insects only. In *R. microplus*, the global research efforts have led to the identification of at least nine mutations (SNPs) in sodium channel gene (Table 12.1). Out of these nine SNPs, four SNPs (T2134A, C190A, G215T, T170C) were non-synonymous and demonstrated to be clearly associated with resistance (He *et al.*, 1999; Morgan *et al.*, 2009; Stone *et al.*2014) and therefore, can be used as molecular markers whereas, five other SNPs {C189A, C2130T (synonymous) C148T, G184C, C190G, (non-synonymous)} did not appear to be associated with resistance or their involvement in conferring resistance remains to be investigated (Stone *et al.*, 2014). Lovis *et al.* (2012) developed a multiplex diagnostic PCR assay that can simultaneously detect the all three known *R. microplus* sodium channel gene mutation (T2134A, C190A and G215T) in one assay. This PCR assay has significantly increased the efficiency of detection of these mutations. Recently, Stone *et al.* (2014) developed three rapid detection assays based on the Melt-MAMA qPCR platform to detect SNPs T170C and C190A in domain II and T2134A in domain III. The development of this qPCR assay for simultaneous detection of more widely distributed resistance associated three SNPs will facilitate high-throughput identification of resistant genotypes in thousand of field ticks within few hours.

Table 12.1: Summary of the Single Nucleotide Polymorphisms (SNPs) Identified in the Sodium Channel Gene in *Rhipicephalus microplus*

Location in Sodium Channel	**Nucleotide Position and Substitution*	*Amino Acid Position and Substitution*	*Reference*	*Notes*
Domain III S6	T2134A	F1550I	He *et al.* (1999)	These four SNPs are already proved to be associated with resistance and can be used as molecular markers for determining resistance
Domain II S4-5 linker	C190A	L64I	Morgan *et al.* (2009)	
Domain II S4-5 linker	G215T	G72V	Jonsson *et al.* (2010)	
Domain II	T170C(Super-kdr)	Methionine/ threonine	Stone *et al.* (2014)	
Domain II	C148T	Leucine/ Phenylalanine	Stone *et al.* (2014)	Further studies are warranted to establish their association with resistance
Domain II	G184C	Glycine/Arginine		
Domain II	C189A	Synonymous		
Domain II	C190G	Leucine/Valine		
Domain III	C2130T	Synonymous		

*All SNP positions numbering corresponding to GenBank accession number AF134316.

Mutation in the Carboxylesterase Gene

Studies of acaricide resistant *R.microplus* ticks have shown that esterases, particularly carboxylesterase (CaEs) is associated with resistance. Hernandez *et al.* (2000) for the first time identified a novel nucleotide substitution of an adenosine (A) for guanidine (G) at position 1120 (G1120A) in CaEs encoding gene of *R. microplus* resulting in the replacement of a amino acid at position 374 from aspartate to asparagine (Asp 374 Asn) (Table 12.2). Although a direct correlation between this mutation and pyrethroid resistance could not be established, this mutation was thought to occur simultaneously with other events that contribute to resistance development (Baffi *et al.*, 2007). This mutation creates an *EcoRI* restriction site (*CTTAAG*) in the mutant individuals and thus its use as a monitoring tool was explored in the form of a polymerase chain reaction-restriction fragment length polymorphism (PCR-RFLP) assay (Baffi *et al.*, 2007; Hernandez *et al.*, 2002). In later studies, this carboxylesterase marker has also found to be associated with organophosphate resistance in *R. microplus* ticks (Baffi *et al.*, 2007; Faza *et al.*, 2013). Nagar *et al.* (2016) did not detect any mutation at position 1120 in the 372 bp CaES gene in reference resistant lines and in any of the field collected *R. microplus* from India. The finding of this study was in contrast to the observations of Hernandez *et al.* (2002), Baffi *et al.* (2007) Chen *et al.* (2009) and recently with Sungirai *et al.* (2018) where the authors utilized the G1120A point mutation to develop molecular tools for rapid detection of pyrethroid resistance in ticks.

Table 12.2: Single Nucleotide Polymorphisms (SNP) Identified in the Carboxylesterase Gene Associated with Resistance in *Rhipicephalus microplus*

*Nucleotide Position and Substitution**	*Amino Acid Position and Substitution*	*Reference*
G1120A	G374A	Hernandez *et al.* (2000)

*A SNP position numbering corresponding to GenBank accession number AF183383.

Apart from target site insensitivity, metabolic detoxification has been implicated in resistance to pyrethroids especially the increased expression of esterase enzymes, which would hydrolyse the acaricide (Rosario-Cruz *et al.*, 2009) and this, cannot be detected by molecular assays. A Tick strain Coatzacoalcos, which is moderately resistant to pyrethroids, the mutation neither in the sodium channel gene nor in the carboxylesterase gene is present, instead, over- expressed esterase activity (a specific esterase designated as CzEst9) which hydrolyzes pyrethroids, believed to be responsible for providing esterase-mediated pyrethroid resistance (Jamroz *et al.*, 2000). This Coatzacoalcos strain makes such an elevated amount of the pyrethroid-hydrolyzing enzyme, CzEst9 (Pruett *et al.*, 2002), that the tick can survive moderate pyrethroid exposure, however, in San Felipe and Corrales isolates that are extremely resistant to pyrethroids, a point mutation in the sodium channel gene (He *et al.*, 1999) is mainly responsible for conferring resistance. Generally, when both mechanisms coexist, target site resistance mechanism plays a more important role.

Resistance Mechanism and Molecular Markers for Organophosphate Resistance

There is probably three potential mechanisms of resistance to organophosphates (OPs): (1) Target site insensitivity in the carboxylesterase gene, (2) Target site insensitivity in the Acetylcholinesterase gene, (3) Metabolic detoxification based OP resistance.

Mutation in the Carboxylesterase Gene

As mentioned in the previous section that the mutation in the CaEs gene has also been associated with organophosphate resistance (Baffi *et al.*, 2007; Faza *et al.*, 2013) and this mutation has played a less significant role in conferring pyrethroid resistance rather than conferring organophosphate resistance in *R. microplus*. Therefore, CaEs gene marker is more useful in diagnosing organophosphate resistance in *R. microplus*.

Mutation in the Acetylcholinesterase Gene

The primary physiological target of organophosphate (OP) and carbamate acaricides is generally considered acetylcholinesterase (AChE), the enzyme responsible for degradation of the neurotransmitter acetylcholine at neural synapses in the central nervous systems of both vertebrates and invertebrates (Fournier and Mutero 1994). Being the target of OP acaricides/insecticides, acetylcholinesterases (AChE) are the enzymes of interest to understand the molecular basis of OP resistance. In *R. microplus,* three AChE genes were characterized as AChE1, AChE2 and AChE3 till date. Baxter and Barker (1998) isolated the first putative AChE gene (AChE1) in *R. microplus* larvae from Australia. Two other putative *R. microplus* AChE genes (AChE2 and AChE3) have since been identified (Hernandez *et al.*, 1999; Temeyer *et al.*, 2004). Point mutations in the gene encoding acetylcholinesterase that result in production of an altered enzyme have been shown to be a major mechanism of OP resistance in several insects like potato beetle, housefly, sheep blowfly (Zhu *et al.*, 1996; Villatte *et al.*, 2000; Chen *et al.*, 2001; Temeyer *et al.*, 2007). Temyer *et al.* (2013) analyzed the sequence data of AChE1, AChE2 and AChE3 genes of nine susceptible and twenty resistant strains of *R. microplus* and identified several amino acid substitutions (Table 12.3) in these genes with variable frequency but due to the presence of multiple copies and transcript polymorphism in each gene, these substitutions were not directly correlated with OP resistance. Due to this reason, molecular genetic markers for OP resistance have been slower to emerge, reflecting a higher degree of complexity of the OP–target–detoxification system (Rodriguez-Vivas *et al.*, 2018).

Although additional factors such as increased expression of AChE, toxin sequestration or metabolic detoxification (Li *et al.*, 2003) may contribute to phenotypic resistance to OP. Increased activity of esterases is one of the most common types of metabolic resistance mechanism found among ticks, mites and insects as it can provide resistance to organophosphates that are esters of phosphoric acid. It is also effective on carbamates due to the existence of ester bonds in their chemical structures (Fukoto, 1990)

Table 12.3: Amino Acid Substitutions Associated with OP-resistance in the AChE Gene of *Rhipicephalus microplus*

AChE1	AChE2	AChE3	Reference
P157S, D188G, E195G, E196G,Y230C, S282G,V331A, T362A, F390S, L417P, Q488R, I493T, P590A, W571R, W571FN566DAmino acid position indicated in GenBank accession number CAA11702	F9L,A26T, E75GW114R, L141F, K208R I210V, K555M, M349VM406V, P343SAmino acid position indicated in GenBank accession number AF067771.	I54V, R86Q, I123MI492M, T548Y,T548AAmino acid position indicated in GenBank accession number AY267337.	Temyer *et al.* (2013)

Mutations in AChE1

A recombinant construct of AChE1 containing several amino acid substitutions was shown to result in a 40-fold reduction in paraoxon sensitivity compared to that of AChE3 of *R. microplus*. Among the 16 amino acid substitutions compared to the susceptible type AChE1 sequence, D188G, E196G, V331A, and F390S were found only in the paraoxon-insensitive construct, and the D188G and F390S substitutions were considered to be most likely candidates responsible for the paraoxon insensitivity (Temeyer *et al.*, 2010) (Table 12.3).

Mutations in AChE2

Ghosh *et al.* (2015) found five new SNPs (G138A, G889A, T1090A, C1234T, G1403A) in the AChE2 gene of laboratory-reared *R. microplus* line IVRI-III and OP resistant field populations, collected from the state of Bihar, India. One of the substitutions (G138A) was a synonymous mutation, while other four nucleotide substitutions were non-synonymous, replace a valine for an isoleucine in position 297 (V297I), a serine for a threonine in position 364 (S364T), histidine for a tyrosine in 412 (H412Y) and a lysine for an arginine in position 468 (R468K). (Table 12.4). They suggested that these mutations could most likely to be associated with OP resistance but as there was a moderate to high range of resistance in the field collected ticks having these mutations, the actual contribution of these mutations in the development of insensitive AChE2 could not been ascertained yet. This can also imply that other factors exist which contribute to insensitive acetylcholinesterase other than point mutations. Nagar *et al.* (2016) studied the role of mutations in AChE2 in the development of OP resistance in *R. microplus* ticks from India. They identified the same four amino acid substitutions (viz. V297I, S364T, H412Y and R468K) in AChE2 gene of resistant field populations and in reference resistant lines of *R. microplus*, as detected earlier by Ghosh *et al.* (2015) (Table 12.4).

Table 12.4: Summary of the Single Nucleotide Polymorphisms (SNPs) Identified in the AChE Gene of *Rhipicephalus microplus*

Targeted Gene	*Nucleotide Position and Substitution*	*Amino Acid Position and Substitution*	*Reference*	*Notes*
AChE2 Nucleotide sequence numbering corresponding to GenBank accession numberAJ278342	G138A*, G889A, T1090A, C1234T, G1403A* synonymous mutation	V297I, S364T, H412Y, R468K	Ghosh *et al.*, 2015Nagar *et al.*2016	Further studies are warranted to establish their association with resistance
AChE3 Nucleotide sequence numbering corresponding to GenBank accession numberAY267337	A366C, A384G, G481AG633A, C1700G, A1866G, T436C, A455G,T459C	I48L, I54V,R86Q, V137I, I492M, T548AV71A, I77M, S79P,	Temeyer *et al.*, 2009Jyoti *et al.*, 2016	

Mutations in AChE3

Temeyer *et al.* (2007) identified six point mutations and their corresponding amino acid change (I48L, I54V, R86Q, V137I, I492M and T548A) in the cDNA sequence that codes for AChE3 in the San Roman strain (OP-resistant strain) of *R. microplus* (Table 12.4). The most frequently occurring mutation was a substitution of glutamine (Q) for arginine (R) at position 86 in AChE3. The role of R86Q was evaluated by expression of the mutant and wild type cDNA sequences in a baculovirus system. Enzyme kinetics of recombinant AChE3 had confirmed that the R86Q mutation increased substrate affinity and conferred insensitivity to paraoxon inhibition (Temeyer *et al.*, 2007). A PCR-RFLP assay was developed to identify the presence of the R86Q mutation in AChE3, which demonstrated that although the R86Q mutation was present at higher frequency in tick strains characterized as OP-resistant, it was also found in OP-susceptible strains indicating that its presence alone was insufficient to produce phenotypic resistance to organophosphate acaricides. This observation was also true of five other reported polymorphisms in AChE3, *i.e.* I48L, I54V, V137I and I492M, T548A (Temeyer *et al.*, 2007; Temeyer *et al.*, 2009; Temeyer *et al.*, 2010). The authors concluded that additional mutations in AChE3, mutations in additional acetylcholinesterase genes, or additional resistance mechanisms (*e.g.* biochemical detoxification mechanism) that contribute to the expression of the OP resistance are likely to occur. Later, in another study, the other five mutations were genotyped and their frequency was evaluated, finding that these mutations were also present in susceptible strains, showing that none of the mutations by themselves is directly responsible for the insensibility of the AChE to organophosphates (Temeyer *et al.*, 2009).

Recently, Jyoti *et al.* (2016) reported six point mutations and their corresponding amino acid change in the AChE3 gene of Indian strains of *R.*

microplus (I48L, I54V, R86Q, V71A, I77M and S79P), in which the first three were previously associated to resistance against OPs in the Mexican San Roman strain (Temeyer *et al.*, 2007) and the other three were reported for the first time. They observed that these mutations are likely to be associated with OP resistance but as the tick strains having these mutations were of varying resistance status (moderate to high), the actual contribution of these mutations in the development of insensitive AChE3 could not be ascertained (Table 12.4).

A considerable number of SNPs and deduced amino-acid replacements were found in the AChE genes of resistant *R. microplus* from different regions of the world. So, the SNPs identified in the resistant strains of *R. microplus* could be classified into two groups. One group includes the major part of reported SNPs, which possibly attributed to geographical population difference because mutations reported from the different strains of *R. microplus*, which were collected from different countries. The others consist of those SNPs, which may contribute to acaricide resistance. However, these mutations need to be further confirmed with site-directed mutagenesis and functional expression experiments.

Resistance Mechanism for Amitraz Resistance

Amitraz is a triazapentadiene compound, a member of the amidine chemical family introduced in 1972. It acts as a non-systemic octopaminergic agonist and has been used for the control of ticks on cattle (Garris and George 1985; Curtis 1985; Kagaruki 1996), dogs and wild animals (Pound *et al.*, 2000; Elfassy *et al.*, 2001; Kumar *et al.*, 2001), parasitic mites of honey bee (Floris *et al.*, 2001), and other ectoparasites of livestock (Curtis 1985). The use of amitraz became more frequent when pyrethroid resistance problems started to hinder the tick control efforts. The first case of amitraz resistance was detected in the San Alfonso strain of *R. microplus* collected from a ranch in the state of Tabasco (Soberances *et al.*, 2002). Reports of resistance against amitraz are available against *R. microplus* ticks from various parts of the world (Jonsson *et al.*, 2000; Li *et al.*, 2004; Veiga *et al.*, 2012; Mendes *et al.*, 2013) and the factors associated with increased probability of *R. microplus* resistance in Australia were identified as region, frequency, doses and application method (Jonsson *et al.*, 2000).

Resistance to amitraz is complex and suggested to be multigenic in nature, involving recessive inheritance of resistance alleles (Li *et al.*, 2004; Li *et al.*, 2005; Fragoso-Sanchez *et al.*, 2011). Till date, no convincing resistance mechanisms against amitraz have been shown for *R. microplus*, but several such mechanisms have been proposed. Bioassay with synergists suggests that metabolic detoxification resistance mechanism through elevated, P450 cytochrome monooxygenases (Ducornez *et al.*, 2005), monoamine oxidase and increased activity of ATP-binding cassette transporters, plays a role in amitraz resistance in some strains of *R. microplus*. (Knowles and Roulston 1972, Li *et al.*, 2004; Lara *et al.*, 2015; Jonsson *et al.*, 2018). Regarding, the molecular basis of target-site resistance, it is thought that amitraz is a potential agonist of the octopaminergic system located in the tick synganglion. It has been suggested that in the presence of amitraz, the octopamine receptor is activated and this overstimulation at synapses has lethal effects on the tick (Lees *et al.*, 2007). The G protein coupled octopaminergic receptors have been classified into three distinct classes, namely α-adrenergic-like octopamine receptor (αAOR), β-adrenergic-like (βAOR), and octopamine/tyramine (OCT/Tyr) or tyraminergic (Evans 2005). The target of amitraz has been proposed to be one of the biogenic amine receptors, most likely the adrenergic or octopamine receptors (Evans and Gee 1980; Hollingworth *et al.*1982).

Baxter and Barker (1999) sequenced the putative octopamine receptor gene from amitraz resistant and amitraz susceptible *R. microplus* Australian strains. Sequence analysis revealed no differentiation between the two phenotypes and thus they concluded that the resistance to amitraz in Australian isolates of *R.microplus* did not appear to be the result of a point mutation in putative octopamine receptor gene. Chen *et al.*, 2007 identified two non-synonymous single nucleotide polymorphisms (SNPs) and their corresponding amino acid substitutions (A22C-T8P; T65C-L22S) that were present in the octopamine/tyramine receptor gene (same receptor as examined by Baxter and Barker in 1999) of amitraz-resistant ticks but not in amitraz susceptible ticks (Table 12.5). However, these SNPs were inferred only by sequence alignment between a susceptible Australian strain, the susceptible American Gonzalez strain, and the resistant Santa Luiza strain (Chen *et al.*, 2007). Both SNPs were in the N-terminal, first extracellular domain, suggesting a possible role for conformational change in the octopamine/tyramine receptor in resistance to amitraz. Earlier studies of the role of the octopamine receptor in amitraz resistance in *R. microplus* (Baxter and Barker 1999; Chen *et al.*, 2007) were not conclusive, but it seems likely that the previous investigations were most likely conducted on an OCT/Tyr-like receptor rather than the native octopamine receptor (Corley *et al.*, 2012). The Mexican Pesqueria tick strain did not show the T8P and L22S mutations (Li *et al.*, 2004) in octopamine receptor gene but confirmed to convey metabolic resistance to amitraz by up-regulation of glutathione-S-transferase (Saldivar *et al.*, 2008). Baron *et al.* (2015) examined the South African field samples of *R. microplus* and demonstrated that the two SNPs were present in the octopamine-tyramine receptor causing amino acid substitutions T8P and L22S, in the resistant samples as previously identified in North America by Chen *et al.* (2007). They demonstrated a very stringent correlation between survival of larvae in the Larval Pocket Tests (LPT) and the genotype. They also designed a RFLP-based assay for genotyping *R. microplus* against amitraz resistance. Robbertse *et al.* (2016) evaluated the acaricide resistance status and the level of genetic diversity in a partially isolated *R. microplus* population in 12 dip stations in South Africa. Approximately half of the ticks sampled proved to be genotypically resistant to amitraz on the basis of the presence of the SNPs described by Chen *et al.* (2007). Very recently, Sungirai *et al.* (2018) found twenty SNPs in octopamine/

tyramine receptor gene of amitraz resistant *R. microplus* tick populations from communal land areas of Zimbabwe. Out of these twenty SNPs detected, eight nucleotide substitutions were similar to those found in the Santa Luisa strain (amitraz resistant) and these included the mutations at nucleotide position 22 (A to C) and 65 (T to C) which are already reported to be potentially associated with resistance to amitraz (He *et al.*, 1999; Chen *et al.*, 2007; Baron *et al.*, 2015). They also used RFLP based assay, designed by Baron *et al.* (2015) to genotype the 367 tick DNA samples and consistently generated six different RFLP profiles. Sungirai *et al.* (2018) also detected an important SNP in resistant samples of *R. microplus* at position 39 and this has been found to be in linkage disequilibrium with the SNP at position 65 (Baron *et al.*, 2015).

Table 12.5: Summary of the Single Nucleotide Polymorphisms (SNPs) Identified in the Octopamine-Tyramine and β-adrenergic Octopamine Receptor Gene (βAOR) Gene of *Rhipicephalus microplus*

Targeted Gene	*Nucleotide Position and Substitution***	*Amino Acid Position and Substitution*	*Reference*
Octopamine-Tyramine	A22C T65C	T8PL22S	Chen *et al.* (2007 Baron *et al.* (2015)
β-adrenergic octopamine receptor (βAOR)	A181T T185C A263C C264A T123C* C126T* A225G* *Synonymous mutation	I61F Isoluecine/Threonine Tyrosin/Serine Tyrosin/Serine	Corley *et al.* (2013 Jonsson *et al.* (2018)

** A SNP position numbering corresponding to GenBank accession number EF490687.

Corley *et al.* (2013) for the first time identified a novel non-synonymous nucleotide substitution of a thymidine (T) for adenosine (A) at position 181 (A181T) in the first transmembrane domain of β-adrenergic octopamine receptor gene (βAOR) of the same amitraz-resistant Ultimo strain of *R. microplus* ticks, as used by Baxter and Barker (Baxter and Barker 1999), which resulted in the substitution of an isoleucine with a phenylalanine (I61F). They found that this particular SNP was only localized to the central Queensland (Australia) region and absent in north and southeast regions, thus minimizing its probability of being the major causative reason for amitraz resistance in Australia. Jonsson *et al.* (2018) have identified seven mutations (SNPs) in βAOR sequences gene of *R. microplus*, collected from diverse locations around the world, including Brazil, Mexico, Australia, Thailand, and South Africa. Out of these seven SNPs, four

SNPs were non-synonymous (A181T, T185C, A263C, C264A) whereas, three other SNPs were synonymous (T123C, C126T, A225G), means no observable substitution effect on the amino acid sequence. (Table 5). Their work has also confirmed the presence of the I61F mutation in amitraz-resistant South American isolates of *R. microplus* and corroborates the belief that variation in βAOR might contribute to resistance to amitraz.

Discovery of diverse mutations only in amitraz-resistant ticks provided the first evidence for the possibility of an altered target site as a mechanism of amitraz resistance in ticks. Amitraz-resistant isolates from Australia and Latin America share mutations in the N-terminal extracellular domain and in the first few amino acid residues of the first transmembrane domain of βAOR. Similarly, amitraz-resistant isolates from the USA, Latin America and South Africa share mutations in the octopamine/tyramine receptor. Given that several mutations have been detected to date and more are possible, the development of a single, comprehensive diagnostic test based on DNA sequence variation alone is likely to be difficult (Jonsson *et al.*, 2018). At present, polymorphisms in octopamine-tyramine receptor and βAOR have some potential for molecular diagnosis of amitraz resistance; however, the diversity of mutations suggests that no single polymorphism can be relied on (Rodriguez-Vivas *et al.*, 2018).

Resistance Mechanism for Macrocyclic Lactone

Macrocyclic lactone (ML) acaricides include the ivermectins and milbemycins. In recent years, ivermectin has emerged as a promising alternative to control tick populations including *R. microplus* resistant to most acaricides. MLs activate glutamate-gated (GluCl) and/or gamma-aminobutyric acid-gated chloride ion channels in nerve and muscle cells in arthropods and nematodes, leading to paralysis of peripheral motor function, inhibition of feeding and reproduction and, ultimately, death (Wolstenholme and Rogers, 2005; Fox 2006). Despite the positive results MLs have afforded in terms of parasite control, the selective pressure caused by the extensive application of these drugs during the past few years has triggered the development of resistance in a number of these parasites, including the nematodes *Onchocerca volvulus* (Townson *et al.*, 1994), *Cooperia spp.* (Coles *et al.*, 2001) and *Haemonchus contortus* (Kaplan 2004; Coles *et al.*, 2005), mites *Tetranychus urticae* (Kwon *et al.*, 2010) and *Sarcoptes scabiei* (Currie *et al.*, 2004), flies *Lucillia cuprina* (Rugg *et al.*, 1998) and *Drosophila melanogaster* (Kane *et al.*, 2000) and cattle tick *R. microplus* and as a result *R. microplus* resistant to ivermectin have been reported in Brazil since 2001 (Martins and Furlong, 2001; Klafke *et al.*, 2006) in Mexico (Perez-Cogollo *et al.*, 2010) and Uruguay (Castro-Janer *et al.*, 2011). At present, the molecular basis of resistance to MLs is not well understood. The insensitivity of the GluCl receptor, which prevents drug binding to its target site, has been associated with ivermectin resistance in some nematodes and arthropods (Cully *et al.*, 1994; Dent *et al.*, 2000; McCavera *et al.*, 2009; Kwon *et al.*, 2010). Recently, it has become evident from several molecular, pharmacokinetic, and biochemical studies that the most important molecules involved in detoxification of MLs are ATP-binding cassette (ABC) transporter proteins (Lespine *et al.*, 2008; Bourguinat *et al.*, 2011). In 2012, Pohl *et al.*, studied the ATP binding cassette (ABC) transporter efflux pumps and their role in ivermectin resistance in *R. microplus*. They studied the transcriptional levels of ABC transporters in the midgut of resistant and susceptible females and found that the ABC transporter efflux pump is a defense mechanism against ivermectin in *R. microplus* and variation in the level of expression of the ABCB10 gene has been associated with resistance to MLs in ticks (Pohl *et al.*, 2012) and to other acaricides using *in vitro* approaches in cell cultures (Koh-Tan *et al.*, 2016). However, despite the evidence of altered ABCB10 expression in resistant populations, the genotypic basis of this variation is not known, and therefore, there are no molecular markers available for resistance monitoring against MLs (Rodriguez-Vivas *et al.*, 2018).

Resistance Mechanism for Phenylpyrazoles

Fipronil is a phenylpyrazolic insecticide, whose mechanism of action is to block insect chloride channels that are controlled by gamma-aminobutyric acid (GABA) receptor in the neurons of the central nervous system (Cole *et al.*, 1993; Bloomquist 2003). Fipronil was initially used to control crop pests as well as other insects of public health importance and was later used to control companion animal ectoparasites (fleas and ticks). This active ingredient began to be used in livestock in the mid-90s for the control of cattle ticks and horn flies (*Haematobia irritans*) (Guglielmone *et al.*, 2000). So far, fipronil resistance has been reported in insects of agricultural and public health importance (MingZhang *et al.*, 2004). Fipronil resistance has also been reported in *R. microplus* from Uruguay (Cuore *et al.*, 2007; Castro-Janer *et al.*, 2009); Brazil (Castro-Jenner *et al.*, 2010) and Mexico (Miller *et al.*, 2013) by different bioassays tests.

Mutation of the GABA receptor associated with fipronil resistance has been reported in the whitebacked planthopper, *Sogatella furcifera* (Nakao *et al.*, 2010) *Drosophila simulans* (Goff *et al.*, 2005) but till date, there have been no reports that show the molecular mechanism of action by which this resistance to fipronil develops in *R. microplus*. The biochemical detoxification mechanism of resistance through enhanced activities of carboxylesterase and microsomal-O-demethylase has also been reported in fipronil-resistant rice stem borer, *Chilio suppressalis* (Li *et al.*, 2007).

Conclusion

The resistance mechanisms for several acaricides that act in the cattle tick *R. microplus* are beginning to be understood at the molecular level. Research is going on to understand the molecular mechanism of resistance that is active in amitraz, fipronil, and macrocyclic lactone resistant *R. microplus*. The development and improvement of DNA based diagnostic tools to identify acaricide resistant *R.*

microplus populations are priorities and in the near future and it will be important to expand the molecular targets involved in acaricide resistance. Such tools will allow control programs to detect and track resistance at an early stage in the field, which is an essential requirement to successfully tackle the growing problem of acaricide resistance in tick control. There is a consensus that the power of whole-genome sequencing to identify genes/regulatory regions that are associated with acaricide resistance would revolutionize the application of molecular markers for rapid and efficient monitoring of acaricide resistance across the tick endemic countries by providing control programs with new markers that predict their impact on resistance phenotypes.

Chapter 13

Monitoring of Acaricidal Resistance with Quantification of "Detoxification Enzymes"

Ashutosh Fular, Nisha Bisht and Srikant Ghosh

Entomology Laboratory, Division of Parasitology,
ICAR-Indian Veterinary Research Institute,
Izatnagar, Bareilly – 243122, Uttar Pradesh

Introduction

The prevalence of life-threatening protozoan diseases in livestock such as Babesiosis, Theileriosis, Anaplasmosis, *etc.* is dependent on the occurrence of their specific vectors. The need to rear crossbred animals for higher milk production, optimum climatic conditions for vectors and lower socio-economic status of the farmers in the tropical country like India, makes it a hub of these diseases. These diseases along with their vectors are responsible for many million losses to the GDP of the country. India, which owns world's largest bovine population of 299.9 million (190.90 million cattle and 108.7 million buffaloes) and also hold record of being highest milk producer in the world, still have lower milk production per capita than other counterpart countries. The losses incurred in the milk and meat production due to chronic diseases, hide or skin loss due to vector bite and economic loss on the treatment of animals has not been analyzed in Indian perspective since 2003. According to Minjaw and Mcleod (2003), about $450 US billion losses are bearded by country due to tick and tick-borne diseases (TTBDs) alone. The control of these protozoan diseases mainly rely on the management of vectors (ticks) responsible for the transmission of the same. The application of chemical acaricides has been the major measure used for the tick control. The ease of application, readily availability and immediate effect of the chemicals had resulted frequent and inadequate use by the owners. The ill management practices along with the selection pressure of the acaricides caused the resistant alleles to flourish in the population and the compounds began ineffective in due course of time. Various resistance reports of organophosphate (OP) and synthetic pyrethroid (SP) compounds against ticks have been published from across the world but the emerging reports of macrocyclic lactones (MLs), fipronil and amitraz has ring an alarming situation for all the researchers associated with these studies. The unavailability of newer compound in reserve and enormous time and fund required for development of another wonder drug is a concern which needs to be address. Surveillance and monitoring of resistance against acaricides is one of the important components of integrated tick management system. For monitoring of resistance, it is necessary to have discriminating concentration (DC) of different acaricides to be tested for resistance characterization. The characterization of acaricidal resistance in ticks started lately in India, with first report of resistance been published in around 2009-10. After establishment of DC of different compounds in IVRI, more than 30 resistance reports from across the country have been reported against several acaricides. In contemporary with the world, recent reports of inefficacy of Ivermectin and Amitraz have been reported from Indian states too.

Mechanism of Acaricide Resistance in *R. microplus*

Resistance to acaricides can be caused by an array of modifications within tick species, namely, behavioural alteration, physiological modifications within the cuticle reducing the acaricide penetration, biochemical changes within the activity of major acaricide detoxifying enzymes, or structural modification within the acaricide target thereby blocking the acaricide binding/action. Overexpression of acaricide detoxifying enzyme classes, such as carboxylesterases (CCEs), glutathione-S-transferases (GSTs), and cytochrome P450s (CYP450) or mixed-function oxidases (MFOs) have been reported to confer acaricide resistance in many populations of insecticide-resistant *R. microplus*. Numerous point mutations conferring target site alteration in voltage-gated sodium channel gene and acetylcholinesterase (AchE) gene have also been identified in *R. microplus*.

Determination of Detoxifying Enzymes

Esterase Assay Procedure

Principle

In this method, α-naphthyl and β-naphthyl ester substrates are hydrolyzed by enzymatic action to alpha-naphthol and β-naphthol which couples to fast Blue (a diazonium salt) forming a diazo dye complex. This diazo dye complex is measured by spectrophotometer.

Procedure

[Ghosh *et al.*, 2017, Fular *et al.*, 2020]

- ☆ Add 20 µl of tick homogenate in adjacent wells in a 96 microtitre plate.
- ☆ Add 20 µl of homogenization buffer in control well.
- ☆ Add 200 µl of working solution of α-naphthyl and β-naphthyl acetate.
- ☆ Incubate the mixtures at room temperature for 15 minutes.
- ☆ Add 50 µl of fast blue solution to each well.
- ☆ Incubated at room temperature for 5 minutes. (Fast blue stain the naphthol produced and SDS stops the reaction)
- ☆ Measure the absorbance at 570 nm in a spectrophotometer.

Monooxygenase Assay Procedure

Principle

The cytochrome P_{450} enzyme also known as monooxygenase. The assay described here does not measure the monoxygenation activity of cytochrome P_{450} enzyme over a substrate, directly, instead it quantifies the total amount of heme content of the larval homogenate and this enables an indirect estimate of the enzyme activity. Hence, the higher the heme content higher should be the enzyme activity.

Procedure

[Fular *et al.*, 2018, Upadhaya *et al.*, 2019, Fular *et al.*, 2020]

- ☆ Add 20 µl of tick homogenate in a 96 microtitre plate.
- ☆ Add 20 µl of homogenization buffer in control well.
- ☆ Add 80 µl of 0.625 M potassium phosphate buffer (pH 7.2) to each well.
- ☆ Add 200 µl of TMBZ solution to each well.
- ☆ Add 25 µl of 3 per cent hydrogen peroxide.
- ☆ Incubate the plates at 5 min in dark.
- ☆ Measure the absorbance at 650 nm.

The Glutathione-S Transferase Assay Procedure

Principle

GST catalyzes the conjugation of L-glutathione to CDNB through the thiol group of the glutathione.

GST + CDNB ⟶ GS-DNB Conjugate + HCl

The reaction product, GS-DNB Conjugate, absorbs at 340 nm. The rate of increase in the absorption is directly proportional to the GST activity in the sample.

Procedure

[Fular *et al.*, 2018, Upadhaya *et al.*, 2019, Fular *et al.*, 2020]

The reaction mixture in each well of the 96 well microtitre plate is prepared as follows:

- ☆ Add 10 µl of tick homogenate in a 96 microtitre plate.
- ☆ Add 20 µl of homogenization buffer in control well.
- ☆ Add 200 µl of working solution in each well as well as in control wells.
- ☆ Incubate the plate for 20 minutes in dark.
- ☆ Measure the absorbance at 340 nm.

Protein Assay

Principle

The principle of this assay is that the binding of protein molecules to Coomassie dye under acidic conditions results in a color change from brown to blue. This method actually measures the presence of the basic amino acid residues, arginine, lysine and histidine, which contributes to formation of the protein-dye complex.

Procedure

- ☆ Add 10 µl of tick homogenate in a 96 wells microtitre plate.
- ☆ Add 10 µl of homogenization buffer in control well.
- ☆ Add 200 µl of Bradford solution in each well as well as in control wells.
- ☆ Incubate the plates for 15 minutes in dark.
- ☆ Measure the absorbance at 595 nm.

Role of Enzyme in Acaricide Resistance in *R. microplus*

The role of enzymes on acaricide metabolism (Schnitzerling *et al.*, 1983; Nolan *et al.*, 1989; Jamroz *et al.*, 2000; Hernandez *et al.*, 2000; Chevillon *et al.*, 2007) is well documented. Of the two broad mechanisms involved in the development of resistance, the role of over-expression of metabolic enzymes on resistance development is established in a number of arthropod species (Hemingway and Ranson, 2000; Rosario-Cruz *et al.*, 2009; Bass and Jones, 2018). The role of GST in the development of resistance to acaricides in *R. microplus* has been documented by different researchers (He *et al.*, 1999; Li *et al.*, 2003; Saldivar *et al.*, 2008). Rosa de Lima *et al.* (2002) used both recombinant and native protein and reported a much higher level of activity in salivary glands than in guts followed by the absence of activity in hemolymph and saliva of *R. microplus* female. The role of monooxygenase in resistance development to pyrethroids in ticks has been reported by several authors. Enayati *et al.* (2010) reported a 6 fold increase in monooxygenase content in resistant populations than that of susceptible Iranian populations of *R. bursa* using 20 larval homogenates as representative samples. Bayugar *et al.* (2008) studied monooxygenases zymograms in the presence of synthetic monooxygenases enzyme substrate in the pyrethroid resistant Mexican tick strain and found three specific polypeptide bands. Densitometric measurement of monooxygenase zymograms showed a statistically significant monooxygenase activity in resistant ticks. Earlier, Enayati *et al.* (2010); Nandi *et al.* (2015); Bandara and Karunaratne (2017); Gupta *et al.* (2016); Yessinou *et al.* (2018); Chigure *et al.* (2018) reported association between over-expression of these enzymes and acaricide resistance in the field populations. It is a well known fact that resistance development involves multiple mechanisms (Baffi *et al.*, 2008; Jamroz *et al.*, 2000; Temeyer *et al.*, 2010; Guerrero *et al.*, 2012). Of the two broadly established mechanisms, the involvement of the metabolic detoxification system (Hemingway *et al.*, 2004) is positively correlated with the development of resistance (Baffi *et al.*, 2008). Irrespective of the substrate for esterases, an elevated activity in laboratory maintained strains (Guerrero *et al.*, 2003; Li *et al.*, 2007; Morgan *et al.*, 2009; Ghosh *et al.*, 2017) and in field isolates (Baffi *et al.*, 2008; Lovis *et al.*, 2012) has given a conclusive evidence of involvement of esterases in SP-resistance. The cytochrome P450-mediated resistance was evidently proved as an important mechanism in four coumaphos-resistant Mexican populations of *R. microplus* (Li *et al.*, 2003). The results suggest the involvement of enzymes in the development of crossresistance to different groups of acaricides. He *et al.* (1999) and Li *et al.* (2003, 2004) reported a significant correlation between elevated expression of GST and resistance to coumaphos, diazinon and amitraz in the *R. microplus* population. Further, Chevillon *et al.* (2007) using DEM as a synergist further demonstrated a direct correlation between overexpression of GST and resistance against deltamethrin in populations of *R. microplus* from New Caledonia.

Dilemma Need to be Resolved

The monooxygenase complex is composed of three key proteins, a cytochrome P450 (CYP), the cytochrome P450 oxidoreductase (CPR) and cytochrome *b*5 and plays a key role in the metabolism and detoxification of xenobiotic substances, including pesticides. In addition, overexpression of these components has been linked to pesticide resistance in several important vectors of disease. Using bioinformatics 115 transcriptomic sequences were analyzed to identify putative pesticide metabolizing CYPs. Cytochrome P450s are a very large and diverse group of enzymes found in all domains of life. They are an extremely important system involved in the metabolism of endogenous compounds and xenobiotics such as drugs, pesticides, plant toxins, chemical carcinogens, mutagens, hormones, fatty acids and steroids. Down- or up-regulation of P450 gene expression can significantly affect the disposition of xenobiotics or endogenous compounds in the tissues of organisms, and thus alter their pharmacological/toxicological effects. In arthropods, an increase in P450 activity is associated with the enhanced metabolic detoxification of insecticides; and a constitutive over expression of P450 genes has been implicated in the evolution of resistance to insecticides and tolerance to plant. The isolation, characterization, classification and nomenclature of specific insect P450s are critical first steps towards understanding their involvement in these important metabolic processes. To date, more than 2000 insect P450s have been recorded in the National Center for Biotechnology Information (NCBI),

Esterases are a group of enzymes that are reportedly associated with acaricide resistance in *Riphicephalus* (*Boophilus*) *microplus*. A comparative analysis was made of the esterase patterns in malathion and deltamethrin-sensitive, tolerant and resistant tick groups, using non-denaturing polyacrylamide gel electrophoresis. Electrophoretical profiles revealed four bands of esterase activity against α-naphthyl acetate; which were dubbed EST-1 to EST-4. The EST-3 and EST-4 were detected in all strains and were classified as carboxylesterases (CaEs). The EST-2, classified as an acetyl cholinesterase (AChE), was detected in all groups, but its staining intensity increased from susceptible to resistant groups, indicating an altered production according to the degree of resistance. EST-1, which was also classified as an AChE, was detected exclusively in tolerant and resistant groups to both acaricides, but displayed greater activity in the malathion-resistant group. These data suggest that these AChEs may represent an important detoxification strategy developed to overcome the effects of acaricides. Glutathione S-transferases (GSTs) are multifunctional enzymes that are responsible for the metabolism and detoxification of both xenobiotic and physiological substances. Metabolism involves the catalysis of thiol additions of the reduced glutathione to organic compounds through their electrophilic centers. The formation of more water-soluble conjugates would facilitate their elimination. The transport of molecules is facilitated by an ATP-requiring active transport system through the multidrug resistance-related protein (MRP).

GSTs act on a wide variety of substrates, and each GST isoenzyme may function very differently from the others, wherein not all GSTs are involved in the detoxification of acaricides. Therefore, it is important to determine the role of the GSTs of ticks in acaricide metabolism. The correlation studies with the enzyme group with the resistance factor obtained in the bioassays is well documented by various researchers. Enzymes inhibitor studies corresponds similar response towards the role played by the detoxifying enzyme as reported in biochemical assays. But the various isoforms of these metabolizing enzymes create a dilemma that which enzyme isoform is actually playing role in the alteration of the susceptibility of these arthropod species. Through standardization of the protocol for the estimation of detoxifying enzyme, a step toward the determination of probable resistance mechanism has already been taken. Still an extensive research is required to know the specific isoforms of enzyme involved. These isoforms detected could be useful in the development of some novel acaricide which will specifically bind to the target enzyme.

Conclusions

The phenomenon of acaricide resistance in ticks has been studied in great detail throughout this decade. Advancements in the form of more sophisticated and precise instruments along with discovery of novel molecular techniques have resulted in increased knowledge on the mechanisms of acaricide resistance occurring in nature. However, the phenomenon of acaricide resistance seems to be mediated by a combination of different mechanisms rather than any single or specific mechanism. Metabolic detoxification through different enzyme groups (CCEs, CYP450s, and GSTs) has been found to be the major resistance-conferring mechanism against all the four acaricide groups in *R. microplus*. More research experiments should be targeted on the accurate identification of up-regulated detoxification genes in acaricide -resistant populations of *R. microplus*. Targeting specific Esterases, Monooxygenases and GSTs that impede the ability of the arthropod to survive acaricide application could be included in the development of a tick control plan. Scientific studies to find out the ways to delay the onset of resistance should be conducted. Also, search for ideas and concepts for environmentally safe vector control strategies should be devised, such as tick control through botanicals, discovery of a novel group of acaricidal compounds with different targets of actions.

REFERENCES

Bandara, K.J., Karunaratne, S.P., 2017. Mechanisms of acaricide resistance in the cattle tick *Rhipicephalus* (*Boophilus*) *microplus* in Sri Lanka. Pestic. Biochem. Physiol. 139, 68–72.

Bass, C., Jones, C., 2018. Editorial overview: Pests and resistance: Resistance to pesticides in arthropod crop pests and disease vectors: mechanisms, models and tools. Curr Opin Insect Sci 27, 4–6.

Bayugar, R.C., Miranda-Miranda, E., Ortiz-Najera, A., Neri-Orantes, S., Olvera-Valencia, F., 2008. Cytochrome P-450 monooxygenase gene expression supports a multi- factorial origin for acaricide resistance in *Rhipicephalus microplus*. Res. J. Parasitol. 3, 59–66.

Chevillon, C., Koffi, B.B., Barré, N., Durand, P., Arnathau, C., De Meeûs, T., 2007. Direct and indirect inferences on parasite mating and gene transmission patterns: pangamyin the cattle tick *Rhipicephalus* (*Boophilus*) *microplus*. Infect. Genet. Evol. 7, 298–304.

Chigure, G.M., Sharma, A.K., Kumar, S., Fular, A., Sagar, S.V., Nagar, G., Upadhaya, D., Saravanan, B.C., Kumar, R., Ghosh, S., 2018. Role of metabolic enzymes in conferring resistance to synthetic pyrethroids, organophosphates, and phenylpyrazole com- pounds in *Rhipicephalus microplus*. Int. J. Acarol. 44, 28–34.

Enayati, A.A., Asgarian, F., Amouei, A., Sharif, M., Mortazavi, H., Boujhmehrani, H., Hemingway, J., 2010. Pyrethroid insecticide resistance in *Rhipicephalus bursa* (Acari, Ixodidae). Pestic. Biochem. Physiol. 97, 243–248.

Fular, A., Gupta, S., Sharma, A.K., Kumar, S., Upadhaya, D., Shakya, M., Nagar and G., Ghosh, S., 2020. Standardization of tick specific biochemical tools for estimation of esterases, monooxygenases and glutathione S-transferase for characterization of acaricide resistance. Pesticide Biochemistry and Physiology, 164, 130-139.

Fular, A., Sharma, A.K., Kumar, S., Nagar, G., Chigure, G., Ray, D.D., Ghosh, S., 2018. Establishment of a multi-acaricide resistant reference tick strain (IVRI-V) of *Rhipicephalus microplus*. Ticks Tick Borne Dis. 9, 1184–1191.

Ghosh, S., Gupta, S., Kumar, K.A., Sharma, A.K., Kumar, S., Nagar, G., Kumar, R., Paul, S., Fular, A., Chigure, G., Nandi, A., 2017. Characterization and establishment of a re- ference deltamethrin and cypermethrin resistant tick line (IVRI-IV) of *Rhipicephalus* (*Boophilus*) *microplus*. Pestic. Biochem. Physiol. 138, 66–70.

Gupta, S., Ajith Kumar, K.G., Sharma, A.K., Nagar, G., Kumar, S., Saravanan, B.C., Gandham, R., Ghosh, S., 2016. Esterase mediated resistance in deltamethrin resistant reference tick colony of *Rhipicephalus* (*Boophilus*) *microplus*. Exp. Appl. Acarol. 69, 239–248.

He, H., Chen, A.C., Davey, R.B., Ivie, G.W., George, J.E., 1999. Identification of a point mutation in the Para-type sodium channel gene from a pyrethroid-resistant cattle tick. Biochem. Biophys. Res. Commun. 261, 558–561.

He, H., Chen, A.C., Davey, R.B., Ivie, G.W., George, J.E., 1999. Identification of a point mutation in the Para-type sodium channel gene from a pyrethroid-resistant cattle tick. Biochem. Biophys. Res. Commun. 261, 558–561.

Hemingway, J., Ranson, H., 2000. Insecticide resistance in insect vectors of human dis- ease. Annu. Rev. Entomol. 45, 371–391.

Hernandez, R., He, H., Chen, A.C., Waghela, S.D., Ivie, G.W., George, J.E., Wagner, G.G., 2000. Identification of a point mutation in an esterase gene in different populations ofthe southern cattle tick, *Boophilus microplus*. Insect Biochem. Mol. Biol. 30, 969–977.

Jamroz, R.C., Guerrero, F.D., Pruett, J.H., Oehler, D.D., Miller, R.J., 2000. Molecular and biochemical survey of acaricide resistance mechanisms in larvae from Mexican strains of the southern cattle tick, *Boophilus microplus*. J. Insect Physiol. 46, 685–695.

Li, A.Y., Davey, R.B., Miller, R.J., George, J.E., 2003. Resistance to coumaphos and dia- zinon in *Boophilus microplus* (Acari: Ixodidae) and evidence for the involvement of an oxidative detoxification mechanism. J. Med. Entomol. 40, 482–490.

Li, A.Y., Davey, R.B., Miller, R.J., George, J.E., 2003. Resistance to coumaphos and diazinon in *Boophilus microplus* (Acari: Ixodidae) and evidence for the involvement of an oxidative detoxification mechanism. J. Med. Entomol. 40, 482–490.

Li, A.Y., Davey, R.B., Miller, R.J., George, J.E., 2004. Detection and characterization of amitraz resistance in the southern cattle tick, *Boophilus microplus* (Acari: Ixodidae). J. Med. Entomol. 41, 193–200.

Nandi, A., Jyoti Singh, H., Singh, N.K., 2015. Esterase and glutathione-S-transferase levels associated with synthetic pyrethroid resistance in *Hyalomma anatolicum* and *Rhipicephalus microplus* ticks from Punjab, India. Exp. Appl. Acarol. 66, 141–157.

Rosa de Lima, M.F., Sanchez Ferreira, C.A., Joaquim de Freitas, D.R., Valenzuela, J.G., Masuda, A., 2002. Cloning and partial characterization of a *Boophilus microplus* glutathione-S- transferase. Insect Biochem. Mol. Biol. 32, 747–754.

Rosario-Cruz, R., Almazan, C., Miller, R.J., Dominguez-Garcia, D.I., Hernandez-Ortiz, R., de la Fuente, J., 2009. Genetic basis and impact of tick acaricide resistance. Front. Biosci. 14, 2657–2665.

Saldivar, L., Guerrero, F.D., Miller, R.J., Bendele, K.G., Gondro, C., Brayton, K.A., 2008. Microarray analysis of acaricide-inducible gene expression in the southern cattle tick, *Rhipicephalus* (*Boophilus*) *microplus*. Insect Mol. Biol. 17, 597–606.

Schnitzerling, H.J., Nolan, J., Hughes, S., 1983. Toxicology and metabolism of some synthetic pyrethroids in larvae of susceptible and resistant strains of the cattle tick *Boophilus microplus* (Can.). Pestic. Sci. 14, 64–72.

Upadhaya, D., Kumar, B., Kumar, S., Sharma, A.K., Fular, A., Bisht, N., Srivastava, S., Boruah, R.R., Nagar, G., Shakya, M., Nath, T. and Ghosh, S., 2020. Characterization of acaricide resistance in *Rhipicephalus microplus* populations infesting cattle in northeastern India and assessment of local plant extracts for tick management. Vet. Parasitol. 277, 109011.

Yessinou, R.E., Akpo, Y., Sidick, A., Adoligbe, C., Karim, I.Y.A., Akogbeto, M., Farougou, S., 2018. Evidence of multiple mechanisms of alpha-cypermethrin and deltamethrin resistance in ticks *Rhipicephalus microplus* in Benin, West Africa. Ticks Tick Borne Dis. 9, 665–671.

Chapter 14

Generation, Curation and Analysis of Bioassay Data for the Identification of Acaricide Resistance

A. Nandi[1], A. K. Sharma, Manisha, S. Kumar, M. Sankar, Nisha Bisht, A. Fular and S. Ghosh

[1]Assistant Professor,
Department of Veterinary Parasitology Faculty of Veterinary Science,
WBUAFS, Kolkata – 37, West Bengal
Entomology laboratory, Parasitology Division,
ICAR- Indian Veterinary Research Institute, Izatnagar,
Bareilly – 243122, Uttar Pradesh

Introduction

The dose–response curve for a target organism usually uses some unit of biological response instead of occupancy of the receptors, on the assumption that biological response relates linearly to receptor occupancy.

Types

a. Conventional Dose-Response Curves
b. Nonmonotonic Dose-Response Curves

- ☆ Determination of LC_{50} value by Probit analysis in MS Excel
- ☆ Observe replication-wise mortality data.
- ☆ Calculate the mean percentage mortality in each concentration

- X is the LC_{95}, it may vary as per acaricide used
- Example is given in Table 14.1.

Table 14.1: Observation of Mortality Data of *in vitro* Bioassay

Conc. (ppm) (X=30 ppm)	*Mortality (per cent)*				
	Replicate 1	*Replicate 2*	*Replicate 3*	*Replicate 4*	*Mean*
x = 30	0	0	0	0	**0**
2x=60	20	20	0	20	**15**
3x=90	40	40	60	60	**50**
4x=120	60	80	60	80	**70**
5x=150	100	100	100	100	**100**

X= LC_{95} of a particular acaricide against reference strain IVRI-I

- **Probit analysis of dose response data (Table 14.1).**

  To perform Probit analysis,
- Transform the concentration into Log values
- Transform the mortality data into Probit values
- If mortality is 0 per cent or 100 per cent, correct it using following formulae and then change it into probit value.

  Corrected mortality for 0 per cent = (0.25/N) x 100

  Corrected mortality for 100 per cent = 1- (0.25/N) x 100

  [Where N is the number of observations in a particular conc.]

%	0	1	2	3	4	5	6	7	8	9
0	—	2.67	2.95	3.12	3.25	3.36	3.45	3.52	3.59	3.66
10	3.72	3.77	3.82	3.87	3.92	3.96	4.01	4.05	4.08	4.12
20	4.16	4.19	4.23	4.26	4.29	4.33	4.36	4.39	4.42	4.45
30	4.48	4.50	4.53	4.56	4.59	4.61	4.64	4.67	4.69	4.72
40	4.75	4.77	4.80	4.82	4.85	4.87	4.90	4.92	4.95	4.97
50	5.00	5.03	5.05	5.08	5.10	5.13	5.15	5.18	5.20	5.23
60	5.25	5.28	5.31	5.33	5.36	5.39	5.41	5.44	5.47	5.50
70	5.52	5.55	5.58	5.61	5.64	5.67	5.71	5.74	5.77	5.81
80	5.84	5.88	5.92	5.95	5.99	6.04	6.08	6.13	6.18	6.23
90	6.28	6.34	6.41	6.48	6.55	6.64	6.75	6.88	7.05	7.33
—	0.0	0.1	0.2	0.3	0.4	0.5	0.6	0.7	0.8	0.9
99	7.33	7.37	7.41	7.46	7.51	7.58	7.65	7.75	7.88	8.09

Transformation of Percentage to Probits

Table 14.2: Example Showing Conversion of Concentration-Mortality Data into Log-Probit Values to Calculate LC_{50} Value

Conc. (ppm) (X=30 ppm)	Log Conc.	Mean Mortality (Per cent)	Probit Mortality
x = 30	**1.477**	0 = 1.25*	**2.74**
2x=60	**1.778**	15	**3.96**
3x=90	**1.954**	50	**5.0**
4x=120	**2.079**	70	**5.52**
5x=150	**2.176**	100 = 98.75*	**7.26**

*Corrected mortality

Now, put the log-probit data in Excel sheet

- ☆ Go to 'Insert' tab
- ☆ Go to Charts
- ☆ Click on 'Scatter'
- ☆ Click on 'Scatter with only markers'
- ☆ A graph will be shown on sheet
- ☆ Right click on any data point on graph
- ☆ A dialogue box will be shown
- ☆ Click on option 'Add trend line'
- ☆ Another dialogue box of will be displayed
- ☆ Click on 'Display equation on chart' and 'Display R-squared value on chart' in 'Trendline option'
- ☆ A trend linear line will be displayed on the graph
- ☆ Now the probit equation (Y=mx + C) is available on the chart to calculate LC_{50} value

Example-

Conc.	Mortality	Log con	Probit Mortality
10	66.667	1	5.430727
12.5	56.111	1.09691	5.153787
20	80	1.30103	5.841621
25	77.143	1.39794	5.74356
50	99.9	1.69897	8.09

For above exampled data, $y = 3.8381x + 1.0663$; $R^2 = 0.8057$

Put the probit value (*i.e.* 5.0) of LC_{50} (50 per cent mortality) in equation

m	*c*	*log con*		*X=(y-c)/m*	*anti-log*
3.8381	1.0663	5	**LC50**	1.024908	**10.5903**
3.8381	1.0663	6.282	**LC90**	1.358811	**22.846**
3.8381	1.0663	6.645	LC95	1.453468	**28.4098**
3.8381	1.0663	7.326	LC99	1.631028	**42.759**

Antilog of x = 10.59 ppm

So, the LC_{50} value is 10.59 ppm

Similarly, LC90, LC95, LC99 also calculated by using Excel sheet.

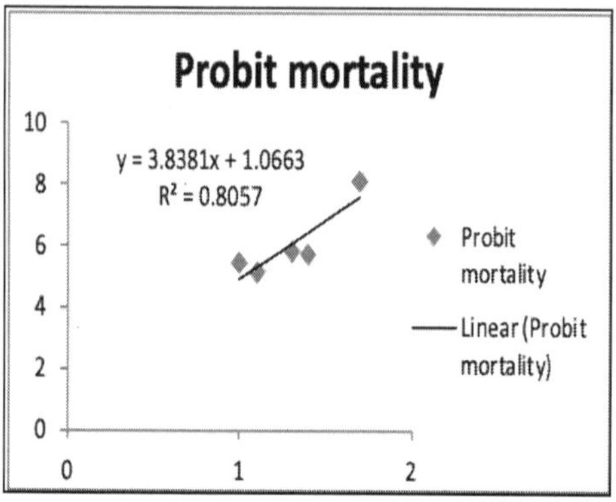

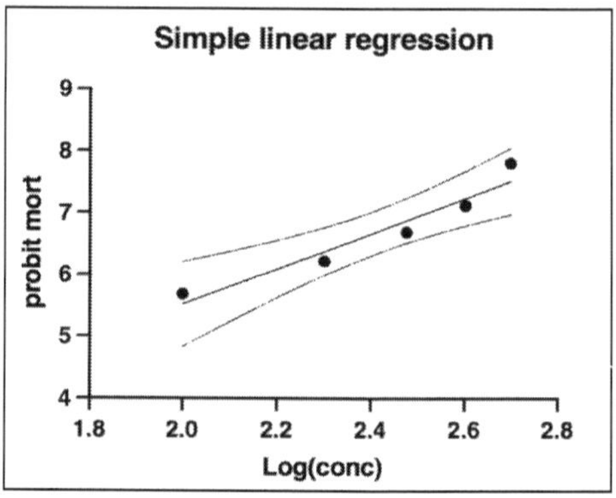

Graph can be Generated by using Excel or GraphPad Prism 9

Determination of Resistance Factor (RF)/Resistance Ratio of field collected ticks

- ☆ LC_{50} and LC_{95} values are calculated by probit analysis of dose response bioassay using 'Microsoft Excel'.
- ☆ The resistance factor (RF) of field ticks is calculated as follows.

$$RR_{50}\ (RF) = \frac{\text{LC50 of acaricide for field ticks}}{\text{LC50 of acaricide for reference susceptible strain}}$$

$$RR95/RR99 = \frac{\text{LC95/99 of acaricide for field ticks}}{\text{LC50 of acaricide for reference susceptible strain}}$$

Calculation of Confidence Interval (CI) of LC50 Value

Calculate LC_{40}, LC_{50} and LC_{60} from linear equation

$S = LC_{60}/LC_{50} + LC_{50}/LC_{40} = \log S\ 2$

Take log value of S

N = no. of ticks used in these 3 concentrations (say 20 in each conc., N = 20+20+20=60, or no. of ticks per conc. x 3)

$$\text{Log f} = \frac{2.77}{\sqrt{N}} \times \log S$$

Take antilog of f (say, 1.05)

Lower limit of CI = LC_{50} value/f value

Upper limit of CI = LC_{50} value/f value

CI = lower limit – higher limit

For Example:

Y = 1.267x + 3.358 (Equation obtained from dose-response curve)

From the above equation,

LC_{40} = 12.5 ppm

LC_{50} = 19.8 ppm

LC_{60} = 31.7 ppm

$$S = \frac{31.7/19.8 + 19.8/12.5}{2} = 1.592$$

Log S = 0.202

N = 20 + 20 + 20 = 60

$$\text{Log f} = \frac{2.77}{\sqrt{N}} \times \log S$$

= 2.77/√60 x 0.202 = 0.0722

f = 1.18

Lower limit of LC_{50} = 19.8/1.18 = 16.8

Upper limit of LC_{50} = 19.8 x 1.18 = 23.4

Thus, Confidence interval = 16.8 – 23.4

Probit analysis of dose IO per cent can be calculated similar way (good correlation found for IVM)

$$\text{Per cent Inhibition of oviposition (IO)} = \frac{\text{RI control} - \text{RI treated}}{\text{RI control}} \times 100$$

Similarly, make a table as follow

Conc.	IO per cent	Log con	Probit IO per cent
10	78.70	1	5.79
12.5	62.34	1.09691	5.31
20	96.38	1.30103	6.92
25	88.36	1.39794	6.18
50	99.9	1.69897	8.09

For above exampled data, $y = 3.5263x + 1.8775$; $R^2 = 0.82$

Put the probit value (*i.e.*, 5.0) of LC_{50} (50 per cent mortality) in equation

Antilog of x = 9.66 ppm

So, the LC_{50} value is 9.66 ppm

Similarly, LC_{90}, LC_{95}, LC_{99} also calculated

Chapter 15

Biological Control Strategies for Acaricide Resistance Mitigation in Ticks

Nirbhay K. Singh, Jyoti and Harkirat Singh

Department of Veterinary Parasitology, College of Veterinary Science
Guru Angad Dev Veterinary and Animal Sciences University,
Ludhiana – 141004, Punjab

Introduction

Ticks are obligate blood-sucking temporary ecto-parasites and transmit a multitude of pathogens affecting both humans and animals. Suborder Ixodida has about 907 different species of ticks, subdivided into 3 families: Nutalliellidae, with a single species, *Nutalliella namaqua*; Argasidae, soft-bodied or soft ticks, with 193 species; and Ixodidae, hard-bodied or hard ticks, with 702 species (Guglielmone *et al.*, 2010). The microclimate along with the abundance and availability of hosts determine the seasonality and prevalence of ticks. In Indian scenario, highly conducive environmental conditions including high ambient temperatures and relative humidity for most parts of year, intensive production system associated endophilous behaviour (restricted to the shelters of their hosts) and negligible active questing increases their chance of survival leading to heavy infestations in field conditions (Singh and Rath, 2013).

Tick infestations cause huge economic losses to the dairy farmers, both directly (by physical effects upon infested animals) and indirectly (through the diseases transmitted) (Ghosh *et al.*, 2007). In India, the annual cost of control of ticks and tick borne diseases (TTBDs) has been estimated at US$ 498.7million (Minjauw and Mc Leod, 2003). Currently, tick control is largely focused on repeated application of chemical acaricides in most parts of the world. However, the indiscriminate and extended use of these chemical acaricides is often associated with serious undesirable effects, such as contamination of milk and meat products with residues, environmental pollution and development of acaricide resistant ticks (Graf *et al.*, 2004). Therefore, alternatives non-chemical strategies including breeding of resistant animals, herbal acaricides, tick vaccines and biological control through pathogens, predators and parasitoids needs to be explored to reduce dependence on chemical acaricides.

Biological Control of Ticks

Biological control is an environment friendly and effective means of reducing ticks through the use of natural enemies or other living organisms as antagonists including predators, parasitoids and pathogens. Predators are generally those free-living species that consume a large number of preys during their lifetime whereas; parasitoids are the species whose immature stages develop on or within the host, ultimately killing it. Pathogens are the disease-causing organisms *viz.* viruses, bacteria, fungi and entomopathogenic nematodes (EPN) which kills or debilitate the host and are relatively specific. Two forms of biological control strategies are generally employed; classical and augmentative bio-control. In classic biocontrol exotic predators or parasites (including parasitoids and pathogens) are introduced to control non-native pest species but has the danger of attacking non-target native taxonomic relatives of the exotic target species (Louda *et al.*, 2005). Whereas, in augmentative biocontrol approach, native predators or parasites are reared in insectaries and released in massive numbers to suppress insect pests (Collier and Van Steenwyk, 2004).

An ideal natural enemy for tick control should have a high fecundity, good searching ability, host specificity and be adaptable to different environmental conditions conducive for its host (tick). High fecundity is most important so that populations of the enemy can rapidly increase when hosts are available. Unfortunately, natural enemies are not very efficient for tick control because their fecundities appear to be far below the level required to respond to the high reproductive rate of ticks leading to explosive increase in numbers. Biological control is becoming an increasingly attractive approach for tick management because of increasing concerns about environmental safety and human health, and increasing resistance of ticks to acaricides. The major groups of tick biological control agents include fungi (*Beauveria bassiana, Metarhizium anisopliae*) EPN (Genus *Heterorhabditis* and *Steinernema*), parasitoids (*Ixodiphagus hookeri*), predators (chicken, Oxpecker) (Samish *et al.*, 2004). The potential of each of these as biocontrol agents is discussed.

Entomopathogenic Fungi

Several species of fungi from the class Deuteromycetes (mitosporic fungi), considered saprophytic organisms and distributed in diverse ecosystems and climates have been reported to interact with arthropods as pathogens (Rajula *et al.*, 2020). The ability of entomopathogenic fungi (EPF) to penetrate the cuticle of tick makes them an effective biological control agent to be included as a component in an integrated tick control strategy (Alonso-Diaz and Fernandez-Salas, 2021). EPF have several advantages over chemical acaricides *viz.* reduction in contamination of milk and meat products with residues, environmental pollution, absence of harmful effects to non-target organisms and short generation interval leading to high production. The most studied EPF worldwide as biological control for ticks in the laboratory and in the field are *Metarhizium anisopliae* and *Beauveria bassiana* mainly against cattle tick, *Rhipicephalus microplus*. EPF have some inherited disadvantages severely affecting their field application as are slow in killing their host, need high humidity to germinate, are susceptible to UV irradiation and some strains are not very host specific (Ginsberg *et al.*, 2002).

Mechanism of Action

The EPF use an entirely different mechanism of action from the chemical acaricides to colonize and kill ticks. They use several invasion mechanisms consisting of enzymatic, toxicological and mechanical systems, which make it difficult for ticks to develop resistance. These fungi target all stages of the tick life cycle (egg, larva, nymph and adults) and could be integrated in control of both on-host and off-host stages of ticks. The EPF infect the ticks in the following sequence of events (Beys-da-Silva *et al.*, 2020):

1. Recognition of the susceptible host
2. Adhesion of conidia and germination on host cuticle
3. Development of specific structures (germ tube and appressorium)
4. Penetration through the host's cuticle
5. Intense fungal growth and death of the host
6. Production of conidia after hyphae emergence through the host cuticle.

The aerial fungal conidia adhere to the host's cuticle through hydrophobic mechanisms primarily mediated by proteins (hydrophobins and adhesions) present on the surface of conidia. Upon attachment they will germinate under optimal conditions producing a germination tube followed by a peg or appressorium for penetration into the host's cuticle (Brunner-Mendoza *et al.*, 2019). The penetration is aided by the production of several hydrolytic cuticular enzymes such as lipases, proteases and chitinases and also mechanical pressure exerted by the appressorium. Once inside the tick, the fungi develop hyphal bodies and blastopores that multiply and disseminate through the hemolymph to invade different tissues for colonization and nutrient absorption causing its death. The fungal toxins (beauvericin, dextruxins) produced act as poisons might cause flaccid paralysis, cellular alterations and inhibit the normal functioning of muscle tissues, the middle intestine and malpighian tubes. Upon tick dead and nutrient depletion, it opens the integument, forms aerial mycelia and carries out sporulation on the corpse, initiating the dispersal of its conidia (Valero-Jimenez *et al.*, 2016).

Entomopathogenic Nematodes (EPN)

The entomopathogenic nematodes (EPNs) are obligate parasite to insects belonging to families, Steinernematidae and Heterorhabditidae and have been successfully used worldwide to control different insect pests (Grewal *et al.*, 2001). *Xenorhabdus* and *Photorhabdus* are bacterial symbionts mutually related to members of families Steinernematidae and Heterorhabditidae, respectively. Steinernematidae has two recognized genera: (1) *Neosteinernema* which comprises only one species, *Neosteinerne malongicurvicauda* and (2) *Steinernema* (type genus) with around 100 recognized species whereas; Heterorhabditidae contains only one genus, *Heterorhabditis* with 20 species (Malan and Ferreira, 2017).

As biological control agent, EPN possess the advantages of having a broad host range and no known negative effect on both environment and non-targeted organisms. They can search and kill their hosts rapidly, are easily mass produced *in vivo* and *in vitro*, are susceptible to genetic selection of desirable traits and are easily applied using conventional equipment. In addition, they can be used with many chemical or biological pesticides or adjuvants (Reis-Menini. 2008). In contrast, their disadvantages are that their broad host range can possibly include beneficial insects, are poorly tolerant to harsh environmental conditions such as soil moisture content, UV radiation and have limited shelf-life.

Tick-Nematode Interaction

Nematodes enter the tick body through natural apertures (engorged *Amblyomma americanum* females) or try to penetrate between mouth parts (*Rhipicephalus* (*Boophilus*) *annulatus*). Ticks can be killed by injection of a single nematode but axenic nematodes (*i.e.* those without symbiont bacteria) are unable to kill ticks hence symbiotic bacteria of nematodes are essential for killing the ticks. A few days after juvenile nematodes penetrate or are injected into ticks, all or most of them die inside their tick host. Although in rare cases they have survived as IJs or even started to develop within the tick, they have not completed their life cycle. However, when the cuticle of ticks was slit artificially before their infection, the nematodes were able to complete their life cycle. Although steinernematids and heterorhabditids infect the ticks in a similar pattern, the steinernematids appear to prefer to search for hosts at or near the soil surface, characterized as ambushers, while the heterorhabditids are adapted to search deeper in the soil and are defined as cruisers (Grewal *et al.*, 2005).

Pathogenicity of EPN to Ticks

The tick susceptibility to EPN infection depends on tick species, stage of tick development, nematode strain and exposure time (Samish *et al.*, 2008).

Studies under laboratory conditions have demonstrated that EPNs represent a promising alternative to develop control strategies for *R.* (*B.*) *microplus* (Singh *et al.*, 2018), *Amblyomma americanum* (Kocan *et al.*, 1998), *R.* (*B.*) *annulatus* (Alekseev *et al.*, 2006), *Ixodes ricinus* (Hartelt *et al.*, 2008) and *Dermacentor nitens* (Monteiro *et al.*, 2014). The use of EPNs against the non-parasitic phase of engorged female ticks can be highly effective, as these engorged females seek environments with high moisture and protected from solar radiation at the time of oviposition, a condition that also favours the survival of EPNs (Grewal *et al.*, 2001).

Heterorhabditids are generally more virulent to ticks than steinernematid nematodes (Goolsby *et al.*, 2018). Fully engorged argasid and ixodid female ticks were generally the most sensitive to EPNs; unfed adult ticks were less sensitive and immature stages the least sensitive, while the eggs were fully resistant (Samish and Glazer, 1991). Different strains or species of IJs have variable influences on the fecundity of engorged females of various tick species and is more pronounced for *Heterorhabditis* strains (Carvalho *et al.*, 2010). Further, EPN exposure also lead to reduced hatchability in tick eggs and may be due its possible deleterious action on the oviposition and/or embryonation process, by interfering in the steps of forming oocytes, fertilization, water absorption by the cuticle and waxing of the eggs by Gene's organ (Silva *et al.*, 2012). Reports indicate that longer exposure times allow a greater number of nematodes to locate and penetrate the host, which apparently increases the effects on the biological parameters of engorged females ticks (Singh *et al.*, 2018).

While feeding on a host, ticks are generally resistant to nematodes except on very moist feeding sites. In a recent study, two EPN species *Steinernema riobrave* and *Heterorhabditis floridensis* were tested for *in-vivo* efficacy against southern cattle fever tick, *R.* (*B.*) *microplus* and caused 14.5 and 25.4 per cent reduction in production of adult engorged female ticks during the first 21 days post treatment. The nematodes significantly affected the reproductive parameters of treated ticks, but not egg hatchability (Goolsby *et al.*, 2018).

Reis-Menini, (2008) reported EPNs particularly *S. glaseri* are compatible with chemical acaricides and can be used together with an organophosphate pesticide for control of ticks in an integrated approach. Recently, efficacy of infective juveniles of several heterorhabditids and steinernematid strains were reported against engorged adult females of the multi-acaricide resistant strain of *R.* (*B.*) *microplus* (Singh *et al.*, 2019). Thus, EPNs might be used as part of an integrated approach to control tick resistant to various classes of acaricides. The EPNs do not undergo their normal propagative cycle within ticks (Zhioua *et al.*, 1995), thereby supporting the hypothesis that ticks are poorer nematode hosts than insects. Nematodes are generally isolated from nature by using insects (larvae of the wax moth, *Galleria mellonelea*) as bait however, in future trials, if ticks are used as bait to attract EPNs in nature, it may be expected that far superior types of nematodes could be isolated for tick control. Therefore, the inclusion of EPNs in an integrated tick-control program can be of immense help and should be considered.

Parasitoids

Most parasitoids used in the biological control of insects belong to the order Hymenoptera and a few species in the genus *Ixodiphagus* of the family Encyrtidae parasitizes ticks (Davis, 1986). The most widespread species is *I. hookeri* (synonyms, *Hunterellus hookeri*) which has been recorded from Asia, Africa, North America and Europe (Hu and Hyland, 1998). Generally, the nymphs are parasitized while they were engorging on vertebrates and development of parasitoid egg is associated with ingestion of blood by tick. The only species that has been released for biological control of ticks is *I. hookeri*. However, it requires high tick densities to persist and is not likely to provide tick control under natural conditions. Nevertheless, inundative releases to control ticks in limited areas (*e.g.* farms, recreation areas) are still potentially feasible (Mwangi *et al.*, 1997).

Predators

Several ants, beetles, spiders and bird species are general predators that occasionally feed on ticks, therefore their populations do not depend on the sizes of the tick populations. General predators can sometimes affect the size of a tick population in nature, but manipulating their populations to reduce tick numbers would require large increases in the predator population, which could also cause large changes in populations of non-target species in natural areas (Symondson *et al.*, 2002).

Birds

Generally thought to be the main predators of ticks and some 50-bird species have been reported to eat ticks (Samish and Rehacek, 1999). Birds either perch on tick-infested mammals or collect them from the ground. Oxpeckers (*Buphagus africanus*: yellow-billed oxpecker and *B. erythrorhynchus*: red-billed oxpecker), both native to Africa, are the only birds that specialize in feeding on ticks. Chickens (*Gallus gallus*) are neither tick-specific predators nor obligatory predators, therefore their consumption of ticks depends largely on alternative food availability and the density of the tick population. Thus, chickens are unlikely to reduce tick densities below a certain level. However, chickens maintained with cattle on small mixed farms can help to reduce tick populations at nearly no additional cost.

Conclusion

Tick and tick-borne diseases are a major concern for sustainable and profitable dairy industry in India. Presently, use of chemical acaricides and systemic acaricides (ivermectin) are the main tick control strategy adopted throughout the country due to absence of any commercialized non-chemical alternate control approach. The problem of tick infestation is basically associated with re-infestation and therefore it is more important to formulate and implement strategies targeting these off-host stages to check re-infestation. The biological control agents like use of EPN, fungi and predators (chicken) in farm which are eco-friendly can easily be used to target these off-host stages and slow down the rate of development of threshold infestations. Although, these biological control agents cannot replace the conventional chemical acaricide but can surely help in reducing the frequency and number of applications by decreasing the off-host tick population.

REFERENCES

Alekseev, E., Glazer, I., Samish, M. (2006). Effect of soil texture and moisture on the activity entomopathogenic nematodes against females *Boophilus annulatus* ticks. *Biocontrol,* **51**: 507-518.

Alonso-Díaz, M.A., Fernández-Salas, A. (2021). Entomopathogenic fungi for tick control in cattle livestock from Mexico. *Frontiers in Fungal Biology,* **2**: 657694.

Beys-da-Silva, W.O., Rosa, R.L., Berger, M., Coutinho-Rodrigues, C.J., Vainstein, M.H., Schrank, A. (2020). Updating the application of *Metarhizium anisopliae* to control cattle tick *Rhipicephalus microplus* (Acari: Ixodidae). *Experimental Parasitology,* **208**: 107812.

Brunner-Mendoza, C., Reyes-Montes, M.D.R., Moonjely, S., Bidochka, M.J., Toriello, C. (2019). A review on the genus *Metarhizium* as an entomopathogenic microbial biocontrol agent with emphasis on its use and utility in Mexico. *Biocontrol Science and Technology,* **29**: 83-102.

Carvalho, L.B., Furlong, J., Prata, M.C.A., Reis, E.S., Batista, E.S.P., Faza, A.P., Leite, R.C. (2010). Evaluation *in vitro* of the infection times of engorged females of *Rhipicephalus* (*Boophilus*) *microplus* by the entomopathogenic nematode *Steinernema glaseri* CCA strain. *Ciência Rural,* **40**: 939-943

Collier, T., Van Steenwyk, R. (2004). A critical evaluation of augmentative biological control. *Biological Control,* **31**: 245-256.

Davis, A.J. (1986) Bibliography of the Ixodiphagini (Hymenoptera, Chalcidoidea, Encyrtidae), parasites of ticks (Acari, Ixodidae), with notes on their biology. *Tijdschrift voor entomologie,* **129**: 181-190.

Ghosh, S., Bansal, G.C., Gupta, S.C., Ray, D.D., Khan, M.Q., Irshad, H., Shahiduzzaman, M., Seitzer, U., Ahmed, J.A. (2007). Status of tick distribution in Bangladesh, India and Pakistan. *Parasitology research,* **101**: S207-216.

Ginsberg, H.S., Lebrun, R.A., Heyer, K., Zhioua, E. (2002). Potential nontarget effects of *Metarhizium anisopliae* (Deuteromycetes) used for biological control of ticks (Acari: Ixodidae). *Environmental Entomology,* **31**: 1191-1196.

Goolsby, J.A., Singh, N.K., Shapiro-Ilan, D.I., Miller, R.J., Moran, P.J., Perez de Leon, A.A. (2018). Treatment of cattle with *Steinernema riobrave* and *Heterorhabditis floridensis* for control of the southern cattle fever tick, *Rhipicephalus* (*Boophilus*) *microplus*. *Southwestern Entomologist*,**43**: 295-301

Graf, J.F., Gogolewski, R., Leach-Bing, N., Sabatini, G.A., Molento, M.B., Bordin, E.L., Arantes, G.J. (2004). Tick control: an industry point of view. *Parasitology* **129**: S427-S442.

Grewal, P.S., De Nardo, E.A.B., Aguillera, M.M. (2001). Entomopathogenic nematodes: potential for exploration and use in South America. *Neotropical Entomology*, **30**: 191-205.

Grewal, P.S., Ehler,s R.U., Shapiro-Ilan, D.I. (2005). Nematodes as biocontrol agents. Wallingford, UK: CABI Publishing.

Guglielmone A.A., Robbins R.G., Apanaskevich D.A., Petney T.N., Estrada-Pena A., Horak I.G., Shao R., Barker S.C. (2010). The Argasidae, Ixodidae and Nuttalliellidae (Acari: Ixodida) of the world: a list of valid species names. *Zootaxa*. **2528**: 1-28.

Hartelt, K., Wurst, E., Collatz, J., Zimmermann, G., Kleespies, R.G., Oehme, R.M., Kimmig, P., Steidle, J.L.M., Mackenstedt, U. (2008). Biological control of the tick *Ixodes ricinus* with entomopathogenic fungi and nematodes: preliminary results from laboratory experiments. *International Journal of Medical Microbiology*, **298**: 314-320.

Hu, R. and Hyland, K. E. (1997). Prevalence and seasonal activity of the wasp parasitoid, *Ixodiphagus hookeri* (Hymenoptera: Encyrtidae) in its tick host, *Ixodes scapularis* (Acari: Ixodidae). *Systematic and Applied Acarology*,**2**: 95-100.

Kocan, K.M., Pidherney, M.S., Blouin, E.F., Claypool, P.L., Samish, M., Glazer, I. (1998). Entomopathogenic nematodes as a potential biological control method of ticks. Ann. *Annals of the New York Academy of Sciences*, **914**: 355-364.

Louda, S.M., Rand, T.A., Arnett, A.E., McClay, A.S., Shea, K., McEachern, A.K. (2005). Evaluation of ecological risk to populations of a threatened plant from an invasive biocontrol insect. *Ecological Applications*, **15**: 234-249.

Malan, A.P., Ferreira, T. (2017). Entomopathogenic nematodes. In. Fourie H, Spaull VW, Jones RK, Daneel MS, De Waele D (eds.), Nematology in South Africa: A view from the 21st century. Switzerland, CH: Springer International Publishing pp. 459-480.

Minjauw, B., McLeod, A. (2003). Tick-Borne Diseases and Poverty. The Impact of Ticks and Tick-Borne Diseases on the Livelihood of Small-Scale and Marginal Livestock Owners in India and Eastern and Southern Africa. UK: Research Report, DFID Animal Health Programme, Centre for Tropical Veterinary Medicine, University of Edinburgh.

Monteiro, C.M.O., Matos, R.S., Araujo, L.X., Perinotto, W.M.S., Bittencourt, V.R.E.P., Dolinski, C., Prata, M.C.A. (2014). First report of pathogenicity of entomopathogenic nematodes of the genus *Heterorhabditis* on partially engorged females of *Dermacentor nitens* (Acari: Ixodidae). *Biological Control*, **69**: 78-81.

Mwangi, E.N., Hassan, S.M., Kaaya, G.P. and Essuman, S. (1997). The impact of *Ixodiphagus hookeri*, a tick parasitoid, on *Amblyomma variegatum* (Acari: Ixodidae) in a field trial in Kenya. *Experimental and applied acarology*, **21**: 117-126.

Rajula, J., Rahman, A., Krutmuang, P. (2020). Entomopathogenic fungi in Southeast Asia and Africa and their possible adoption in biological control. *Biological control*,**151**: 104399.

Reis-Menini, C.M.R., Prata, M.C.A., Furolng, J., Silva, E.R. (2008). Compatibility between the Entomopathogenic nematode *Steinernema glaseri* (Rhabditida: Steinernematidae) and an acaricide in the control of *Rhipicephalus* (*Boophilus*) *microplus* (Acari: Ixodidae). *Parasitology Research*, **103**: 1391-1396.

Samish, M., Ginsberg, H., Glazer, I. (2008). Anti-tick biological control agents: assessment and future perspectives. In: Bowman, A.S., Nuttall, P.A. (Eds.), Ticks: Biology, Disease and Control. Cambridge University Press, Cambridge, pp. 447–-469.

Samish, M., Glazer, I. (1991). Killing ticks with parasitic nematodes of insects. *Journal of invertebrate pathology*, **58**: 281-282.

Samish, M. and Rehacek, J. (1999). Pathogens and predators of ticks and their potential in biological control. *Annual review of entomology*, **44**: 159-182.

Samish, M., Ginsberg, H., Glazer, I. (2004). Biological control of ticks. *Parasitology*. **129**: S389-S403.

Silva, E.R., Monteiro, C.M.O., Reis-Menini, C., Prata, M.C.A., Dolinski, C., Furlong, J. (2012). Action of *Heterorhabditis indica* (Rhabditida: Heterorhabditidae) strain LPP1 on the reproductive biology of engorged females of *Rhipicephalus microplus* (Acari: Ixodidae). *Biological Control*, **62**: 140-143.

Singh, N.K., Goolsby, J.A., Shapiro-Ilan, D.I., Miller, R.J., Thomas, D.B., Klafke, G.M., Tidwell, J.P., Racelis, A.E., Grewal, P.S., Perez de Leon, A.A. (2018). Efficacy evaluation of six entomopathogenic nematode species against engorged females of southern cattle fever tick, *Rhipicephalus* (*Boophilus*) *microplus*. Southwest *Southwestern Entomologist*, **43**: 1-17.

Singh, N.K., Goolsby, J.A., Jyoti, Shapiro-Ilan, D.I., Miller, R.J., Perez de Leon, A.A. (2019). Comparative efficacy of entomopathogenic nematodes against a multiacaricide resistant strain of southern cattle fever tick, *Rhipicephalus microplus*. *Southwestern Entomologist*, **44**: 143-153.

Singh, N.K., Rath, S.S. (2013). Epidemiology of ixodid ticks in cattle population of various agro-climatic zones of Punjab. *Asian Pacific journal of tropical medicine*, **6**: 947-951.

Symondson, W.O.C., Sunderland, K.D. and Greenstone, M.H. (2002). Can generalist predators be effective biocontrol agents? *Annual review of entomology*, **47**: 561-594.

Valero-Jiménez, C.A., Wiegers, H., Zwaan, B.J., Koenraadt, C.J., van Kan, J.A. (2016). Genes involved in virulence of the entomopathogenic fungus *Beauveria bassiana*. *Journal of Invertebrate Pathology*, **133**: 41-49.

Zhioua, E., Lebrun, R.A., Ginsberg, H.S., Aeschllimann, A. (1995). Pathogenicity of *Steinernema carpocapsae* and *S. glaseri* (Nematoda: Steinernematidae) to *Ixodes scapularis* (Acari: Ixodidae). *Journal of medical entomology*, **32**: 900-905.

Chapter 16

Development of Phytoacaricide Formulations for the Control of Acaricide Resistance in Ticks

Reghu Ravindran

Department of Veterinary Parasitology,
College of Veterinary and Animal Sciences,
Kerala Veterinary and Animal Sciences University, Pookode,
Lakkidi, P.O., Wayanad – 673576, Kerala

Introduction

The reports on the resistance of ticks to chemical acaricides are in the increasing trend. After the first report of resistance of *Rhipicephalus microplus* to BHC (Chaudhuri and Naithani, 1964). Large number of reports were published from different parts of the country on the resistance against different acaricides. More reports were from northern India *viz.*, Jammu and Kashmir, Uttar Pradesh, Uttarakhand, Haryana, Rajasthan, Gujarat, Punjab, Bihar while a few reports were published from southern India too *viz.*, Andhra Pradesh, Kerala. Hence, there is an urgent need for evolving newer strategies for the effective and eco-friendly tick control in the country. Many reviews focus on the different aspects of the tick control in the backdrop of acaricidal resistance (Ghosh *et al.*, 2007; Ghosh and Nagar, 2014; Mondal *et al.*, 2013; Kumar *et al.*, 2021). Among the techniques used for the tick control, one of the most promising methods is the development of acaricides of herbal origin. The crude herbal formulations, their fractions or phytochemical compounds may be identified, formulated, and validated for the control of ticks.

The natural products are always considered as alternative to synthetic chemical acaricides, since the secondary metabolites present in the plants protect the plants from the invading microorganisms and arthropods. The secondary metabolites are competitive weapons against other living things such as animals, plants, insects, and microorganisms. The secondary metabolites can target the parasites by different routes. They can attack the nucleic acid (DNA or RNA), cell membrane, cytoskeleton or nervous system. The DNA alkylating compounds cause intercalation and affect the DNA replication process. The alkaloids perform DNA alkylation. Some examples include furanoquinoline alkaloids, pyrrolizidine alkaloids, and furanocoumarins. Another mechanism by which the nucleic acid is affected is based on the inhibition of the enzyme DNA topoisomerase I or II that are essential for the replication process. The cells treated with alkylating and intercalating drugs or topoisomerase inhibitors usually undergo programmed cell death by apoptosis (Wink, 2012).

The actin filaments and microtubules are very important constituents of parasite cytoskeleton. The compounds that can inhibit the polymerisation of tubulin into microtubules (Colchicine, Vinblastine) or inhibit the depolymerization of microtubules (Paclitaxel) can cause damage to the cells (Wink, 2012). The biomembranes of cells function as permeation barrier to prevent the escape of cellular metabolites. They prevent the uncontrolled entry of polar or toxic exogenous the compounds. If fluidity or permeability of the biomembrane is disturbed by compounds with detergent properties, they can cause cytotoxic or antimicrobial effects.Triterpenoid and steroidal saponins can exert cell death by this mechanism (Wink, 2012).

Multicellular parasites have a nervous system with a number of important neurotransmitter/neuroreceptor systems (*e.g.*, acetyl choline receptors) or ion channels (sodium channels).When the neurotransmitter/neuroreceptor systems are inhibited or overstimulated, muscular paralysis will result. Muscular paralysis will also occur if sodium and potassium channels are either blocked or stimulated, because ion signaling is essential in neuronal activity. The alkaloids have neurotoxic properties; they act as agonists or antagonists at neuroreceptors and/or ion channels (Wink, 2012).

The secondary metabolites of plants (Thirumurugan *et al.*, 2012) are classified into five main classes,

- Terpenoids and steroids: They are derived from isopentenyl diphosphate (IPP). Steroids have common tetracyclic carbon skeleton and are modified terpenoids that are biosynthesized from the triterpene lanosterol.
- Fatty acid-derived substances: Biosynthesized from simple acyl precursors such as propionyl CoA, acetyl CoA, and methyl malonyl CoA.

- ☆ Polyketides, alkaloids: A basic structure of alkaloids consists of basic amine group and is derived biosynthetically from amino acids.
- ☆ Non-ribosomal polypeptides: These amino acids derived compounds are biologically synthesized by a multifunctional enzyme complex without direct RNA transcription.
- ☆ Enzyme cofactors: Nonprotein, low-molecular enzyme components

Among the secondary metabolites of plants, tannins are water soluble polyphenols having antimicrobial effects. The flavonoids are also plant secondary metabolites having polyphenolic structure, widely found in fruits, vegetables and certain beverages. They may or may not be water soluble. The flavonoids are again classified into isoflavones, neoflavanoids, flavones, flavanols, flavanones, flavanonols, flavanols or catechins, anthocyanins and chalcones (Panche *et al.*, 2016). Terpenes are simple hydrocarbons and are commercially important fragrance and flavoring agents. Terpenoids are divided into monoterpenes, sesquiterpenes, diterpenes, sesterpenes, and triterpenes depending on its carbon units.

Alkaloids are a group of naturally occurring organic compounds which contain nitrogen atom or atoms (amino or amido in some cases) in their structures. These nitrogen atoms cause alkalinity of these compounds. These nitrogen atoms are usually situated in some ring (cyclic) system. For example, indole alkaloids are those that contain nitrogen atom in indole ring system. Other classification system is connected with the family of plant species from which they are isolated. *e.g.*, opium alkaloids that occur in the opium poppy (Kurek, 2019).

The development of a phytoacaricide include many steps

1. Colonisation of ticks
2. Standardization of bioassay
3. Preparation of crude extracts
4. Fractionation of effective crude extract
5. Chromatography
6. Identification of possible lead phytoacaricide molecules
7. *In vitro* testing
8. *In vivo* validation
9. Development of formulation
10. Identification of mode of action
11. Field validation
12. Multilocation trials
13. Bulk production

Both resistant and non-resistant colonies of single and multi-host ticks can be maintained. The maintenance of tick colony is highly labour intensive procedure. The permission from institutional animal ethics committee (IAEC) and committee for the control and supervision of experimentation in animals (CCSEA) are essential for rearing of animals for the experimentation in India. One host ticks can be colonised in calves (*Rhipicephalus annulatus*) while for developing multihost tick colony (*Haemaphysalis bispinosa*), rabbits and calves can be employed. The fully engorged ticks dropped from the animals are used for the bioassay (adult immersion test).

Immediately upon arrival at the laboratory, the engorged female ticks should be washed, preferably in distilled water, to remove any eggs laid during transport. The engorged female ticks can be refrigerated for five days without adverse effects on their response to adult immersion test (AIT) if stored immediately after detachment. Those ticks that have already started egg lay may not be used for AIT. For all ixodid ticks, the incubation conditions for engorged female ticks, eggs and larvae before testing should be 27 to 28°C and 85 to 95 percent relative humidity (RH). The adult immersion test (AIT) described by Drummond *et al.* (1973) is used to determine the relative effectiveness of the new developed acaricides against a number of tick species.

The plant used for the extraction may be identified with the help of a botanist. A herbarium may be prepared and deposited in the repository for getting the accession number. The plant (leaves, seeds, aerial parts *etc.*) may be collected, dried under the shade and pulverised. The crude extraction may be performed with the help of ethanol as the solvent using a Soxhlet apparatus. The solvent recovery may be performed using a rotavapor. The acaricidal effects of the plant extract may be evaluated based on the mortality of adult ticks, inhibition of fecundity and prevention of hatching of eggs laid by the treated ticks. The crude extract may be dissolved in another solvent which is having minimum acaricidal effects (Ravindran *et al.*, 2011a, b, c). Once the crude extracts are identified as acaricidal (Ravindran *et al.*, 2011d, 2012, 2015, 2017b; Juliet *et al.*, 2012; Sunil *et al.*, 2013; Palayullaparambil *et al.*, 2016; Udayan *et al.*, 2020), they may be used for fractionation using solvents of ascending polarity. The fractions may be further sub-fractionated using column chromatography or flash chromatography. The different fractions and subfractions may also be tested for their acaricidal effects (Krishna *et al.*, 2014; Nair *et al.*, 2017; Divya *et al.*, 2014,2019; Ramachandran *et al.*, 2021; Ravindran *et al.*, 2017a). After ascertaining the acaricidal effects, the subfractions may be evaluated further for their chemical composition using GCMS or LCMS. The identified compounds may also be tested for their acaricidal effects. The phytochemical compounds finally identified may be used for the development of the acaricidal formulation. The formulation may also be tested *in vitro* (Ravindran *et al.*, 2017b) followed by *in vivo*. These validated formulations may be evaluated for their acaricidal activity on infested animals of different geoclimatic conditions before developed into a product for use by farmers.

REFERENCES

Chaudhuri, R.P., Naithani, R.C., 1964. Resistance to BHC in the cattle tick *Boophilus microplus* (Can.) in India. Bull. Entomol. Res. 55, 405–410.

Divya, T. M., Soorya, V. C., Amithamol, K. K., Juliet, S., Ravindran, R., Nair, S. N., Ajithkumar, K. G. 2014. Acaricidal activity of alkaloid fractions of *Leucas indica* Spreng against *Rhipicephalus* (*Boophilus*) *annulatus* tick. Tropical Biomedicine, 31, 46-53.

Divya, T. M., Soorya, V. C., Amithamol, K.K., Udayan, D., Sreelekha, K., Nair, S. N., Ajithkumar, K. G., Juliet, S., Ravindran, R., Ghosh,S. 2019. Acaricidal activity of crude ethanolic extract of *Sphaeranthus indicus*, its fractions and subfractions against *Rhipicephalus* (*Boophilus*) *annulatus* (Acari: Ixodidae). International Journal of Current Microbiology and Applied Sciences 8, 787-797.

Ghosh, S., Azhahianambi, P., Yadav, M.P., 2007. Upcoming and future strategies of tick control: a review. Journal of Vector Borne Diseases 44,79-89.

Ghosh, S., Nagar, G., 2014. Problem of ticks and tick-borne diseases in India with special emphasis on progress in tick control research: A review. Journal of Vector Borne Diseases 51, 259-270.

Juliet, S., Ravindran, R., Sunil, A. R., Kumar, K. G.A., Nair, S. N., Amithamol, K. K., Bandyapadhyay, A., Rawat, A. K. S., Ghosh, S. 2012. *Jatropha curcass* (Linn) leaf extract –a possible alternative for population control of *Rhipicephalus* (*Boophilus*) *annulatus*. Asian Pacific Journal of Tropical Disease, 2, 225-229.

Krishna, T. P. A., Krishna, T. P. A., Chitra, N. D., Deepa, P. E., Udayan, D., Sreelekha, K. P., Juliet, S., Nair, S. N., Ravindran R., Ajithkumar, K. G., Ghosh, S. 2014. Acaricidal activity of petroleum ether extract of *Tetrastigma leucostaphylum* (Dennst.) Alston against *Rhipicephalus* (*Boophilus*) *annulatus*. The Scientific World Journal, Article ID: 715481, http: //dx.doi.org/10.1155/2014/715481

Kumar, R., Sharma, A.K., Ghosh, S., 2020. Menace of acaricide resistance in cattle tick, *Rhipicephalus microplus* in India: Status and possible mitigation strategies. Veterinary Parasitology 278,108993

Kurek, J. 2019. Alkaloids - Their Importance in Nature and for Human Life. DOI: 10.5772/intechopen.85400http: //dx.doi.org/10.5772/intechopen.85400

Mondal, D.B., Sarma, K., Saravanan, M., 2013. Upcoming of the integrated tick control program of ruminants with special emphasis on livestock farming system in India. Ticks and Tick-Borne Diseases, 4, 1-10.

Nair, S.N., Juliet, S., Amithamol, K.K., Sunil,A.R., Palayullaparambil, A.K.T., Sreelekha,K., Divya, T.M., Udayan,D., Kumar, K.G.A., Ghosh, S., Ravindran, R. 2017. *In vitro* acaricidal effects of ethanolic extract and its fractions of

Ageratum conyzoides L. against common cattle tick *Rhipicephalus* (*Boophilus*) *annulatus*. Annals of Phytomedicine 6, 162-16

Palayullaparambil, A. K. T., Palayullaparambil, A. K. T., Juliet, S., Renganathan, K., Raju, R., Athalathil, S., Ravindran, R., Chandrashekar, C., Nair, S.N., Ghosh, S., 2016. Pharmaco-chemical characterization and acaricidal activity of ethanolic extract of *Chassalia curviflora* (Wall ex Kurz.) Thwaites. Pharmacognosy Journal 8, 215-219

Panche, A., Diwan, A., Chandra, S. 2016. Flavonoids: An overview. Journal of Nutritional Science,5,E47 doi: 10.1017/jns.2016.41

Ramachandran, P.D., Muniyappa, M.D., Kanapadinchareveetil, S.,Nair, S.N., Ajithkumar, K.G., Samraj, S., Rajappan, A., Varghese, A., Kalarickal, D.C., Ravindran, R., Ghosh, S., Juliet, S. 2021. Modulation of the PGE2-Mediated Pathway in the eclosion blocking effect of flumethrin and terpenoid subfraction isolated from *Artemesia nilagirica* in *Rhipicephalus annulatus*. Molecules, 26, 4905.

Ravindran, R., Juliet, S., Ajith Kumar, K. G., Sunil, A. R., Amithamol, K. K., Nair, S. N., Chandrasekhar, L., Sujith, S., Bandyapadhyaya, A., Rawat, A. K. S., Ghosh, S. 2011a. Effect of solvents and surfactants against *Haemaphysalis bispinosa*. Tropical Biomedicine, 28,482-486.

Ravindran, R., Juliet, S., Kumar, K. G.A., Amithamol, K. K., Sunil, A. R., Nair, S. N., Priya, M. N., Ghosh, S. 2011b.Toxicity of DMSO, Triton X-100 and Tween 20 against *Rhipicephalus* (*Boophilus*) *annulatus*. Journal of Parasitic Diseases, 35, 237-239.

Ravindran, R., Juliet, S., Kumar, K.G.A., Sunil, A.R., Nair, S.N., Amithamol, K.K., Rawat, A. K. S., Ghosh,S. 2011c.Toxic effects of various solvents against *Rhipicephalus* (*Boophilus*) *annulatus* Ticks and Tick-borne Diseases 2,160– 162

Ravindran, R., Juliet, S., Sunil, A. R., Kumar, K. G. A., Nair, S. N., Amithamol, K. K., Shynu, M., Rawat, A. K. S., Ghosh, S. 2011d. Eclosion blocking effect of ethanolic extract of *Leucas aspera* (Lamiaceae) *on Rhipicephalus* (*Boophilus*) *annulatus*. Veterinary Parasitology 179, 287-290.

Ravindran, R., Juliet, S., Sunil, A. R., Ajith Kumar, K. G., Nair, S. N., Amithamol, K. K., Bandyopadhyay, A., Rawat, A. K. S., Ghosh, S. 2012. Acaricidal activity of *Cassia alata* against *Rhipicephalus* (*Boophilus*) *annulatus*. Experimental Applied Acarology, 56, 69-74.

Ravindran, R., Chithra, N. D., Deepa, P. E., Juliet, S., Kumar, K.G.A., Nair, S.N., Udayan, D., Nanjundappa, S., Chandrasekhar, L., Ghosh, S. 2015. Contrasting effects of ethanolic extracts of leaf and flower of *Chromolaena odorata* against *Rhipicephalus* (*Boophilus*) *annulatus*. Indian Journal of Animal Sciences, 85, 844–848

Ravindran, R., Chithra, N.D., Deepa, P.E., Ajithkumar, K.G., Chandrasekhar, L., Sreelekha, K., Nair, S.N., Juliet, S. and Ghosh, S.2017a. *In vitro* effects of caffeic acid, nortriptyline, precocene I and quercetin against *Rhipicephalus annulatus* (Acari: Ixodidae). Experimental and Applied Acarology, 71, 183-193.

Ravindran, R., Juliet, S., Ramankutty, S. A., Sathish, N., Nair, S. N., Ajithkumar, K. G., Chandrasekhar, L., Ghosh, S. 2017b. Effects of ethanolic extract of the leaves of *Pongamia glabra* and *Gliricidia sepium* against *Rhipicephalus (Boophilus) annulatus*. Advances in Animal and Veterinary Sciences 5: 1-6.

Sunil, A. R., Amithamol, K. K., Juliet, S., Nair, S. N., Kumar, K. G. A., Soorya V. C., Divya, T. M., Jyothimol, G., Ghosh, S., Ravindran, R. 2013. Acaricidal effect of *Cassia fistula* Linn. leaf ethanolic extract against *Rhipicephalus (Boophilus) annulatus*. Tropical Biomedicine, 30: 231-237.

Thirumurugan, D., Cholarajan, A., Raja, S.S.S., Vijayakumar, R.2018. Secondary Metabolites. DOI: 10.5772/intechopen.79766.

Kumar, R., Sharma, A.K., Ghosh, S. 2020. Menace of acaricide resistance in cattle tick, *Rhipicephalus microplus* in India: Status and possible mitigation strategies. Veterinary Parasitology 278,108993

Udayan, D., Nair, S. N., Juliet, S., Ravindran, R., Athalathil, S., Adarshkrishna, T. P., Ajithkumar, K. G., Sreelekha, K. P., Chandrasekahar, L., Ghosh, S. 2020. Acaricidal activity of *Artemisia nilagirica* leaves against *Rhipicephalus (Boophilus) annulatus* ticks. Planta Medica 86, 1335-1344.

Wink, M. 2012. Medicinal Plants: A Source of Anti-Parasitic Secondary Metabolites Molecules 17, 12771-12791 DOI: 10.5772/intechopen.79766

Chapter 17

Problems in Development of Suitable Vaccine against Multi-Tick Infestation in India

H.V. Manjunathachar[1] *and S. Ghosh*

[1]*ICMR-National Animal Resource Facility for Bio-Medical Research, Genome Valley, Shamirpet, Hyderabad – 500101, Telangana*
ICAR-Indian Veterinary Research Institute, Izatnagar, Bareilly – 243122, Uttar Pradesh

Introduction

Ticks are obligate hematophagous ectoparasites, responsible for the transmission of viral, bacterial, and protozoal diseases of man and animals and also produce significant economic losses to cattle industry. As vectors, ticks rank second next to mosquitoes for many human pathogens and first for vector borne diseases of domestic and companion animals. They are considered to be a most competent and versatile vectors due to their wide host range and tendency to feed on several hosts during their life cycle, enable them to acquire and transmit infectious organisms (Jongejan *et al.*, 2004). Globally, 914 tick species are indentified so for and out of these, 106 tick belonging to Argasidae and Ixodidae were documented from India (Geevarghese *et al.*, 1997; Burger *et al.*, 2014). Approximately eighty per cent of the world's tick fauna are Ixodid ticks (Hard ticks- 683 species). The remaining are Argasid ticks (soft ticks-183 species). In addition, the family Nuttalliellidae contains only one species (Jongejan and Uilenberg, 2004). Among three families, the argasid and ixodid ticks are of greater veterinary and medical importance. The geographic distribution and vector capacity of each tick species depends upon its environmental conditions and biotopes (de la faunte *et al.*, 2017).

Incidences of tick-borne diseases (TBDs) are increasing day by day insidiously due to influence of several biotic and abiotic factors, which includes global warming, environmental and ecological changes, and availability of suitable habitats. A report by Centers for Disease Control and Prevention (CDC) shows that, the incidence of TBD's has increased two folds since year 2005 (Rosenberg *et al.*, 2018; de la faunte, 2018). Ticks have a great impact on public health due to several human diseases transmitted by them like lyme borreliosis, anaplasmosis, babesiosis, ehrlichiosis, Crimean-Congo Haemorrhagic Fever (CCHF), Kyasanur forest disease (KFD), Omsk hemorrhagic fever virus, Powassan encephalitis virus and many other rickettisial diseases are increasingly gaining more attention from public health experts, across the world (de la faunte, 2017; Paules *et al.*, 2018). Tick borne diseases (TTBDs) are also ranked high in terms of their impact on the livelihood of resource poor farming communities in developing countries (Perri*et al.*, 2002; Minjauw and McLeod, 2003).

Even though, integrated pest management (IPM) programme was introduced in 1960 chemicals (acaricides) remain the frontline tool for control of economically important arthropods including ticks (Taylor, 2001; Ostfeld*et al.*, 2006). Repeated application of chemical acaricides belongs to different class *viz.*, arsenicals, organchlorines, organophosphates, carbamates, synthetic pyrethroids and avermectins/milbemycins are the most common method adopted by the cattle owners throughout the world. However, the continuous and indiscriminate use of acaricides results in increasing in acaricide tick resistance, acaricide residue accumulation in meat, milk, and the environment.

In India, survey on acaricide resistance conducted through questionnaire reported the possibility of development of large-scale acaricide resistance in India (FAO, 2004). However, the experimental data on acaricide resistant status in Indian ticks was reported against diazinon resistance (Kumar *et al.*, 2011). Subsequently, resistance monitoring tools have been standardized and a large scale development of resistance in Indian ticks against deltamethrin, cypermethrin (Sharma *et al.*, 2012; Shyma *et al.*, 2012) and Amitraz (Singh *et al.*, 2013; Kumar *et al.*, 2014) has been reported. According to Whalon *et al.* (2008), *Rhipicephalus microplus* developed resistance to almost every class of chemical registered for use against it and ranked sixth amongst the resistant arthropods. Regardless of the demonstrated success of acaricides, societal and scientific concerns over the exclusive dependency upon chemicals have emphasized the need for the development and introduction of alternatives to acaricides that are consistent with the principles of sustainable IPM concept. Further, development of next generation acaricides to combat rapid acaricide resistance in ticks fetches heavy cost (de la Fuente and Kocan, 2006). On an estimate, the cost for discovering and developing a noble chemical product is around US$ 100 million, with an average duration of 10 years (Graf *et al.* (2004).

These issues enforced the scientific community to develop and introduce alternatives to acaricides that are consistent with the principles of sustainable TTBDs control. The alternative approaches are strategic use of a number of components *viz.*, use of hosts naturally resistant to ticks, strategic use of effective acaricides, use of resistance monitoring system for identification of zone specific effective acaricides, botanical (herbal) acaricides and repellents, pheromone-impregnated decoys for attracting and killing ticks, biological control method, education about recommended practices to reduce exposures to ticks and development of anti-tick vaccination. Relative to the other alternative methods, the immunological tick control is regarded as a user-friendly and sustainable treatment method (Willadsen, 2006; de la Fuente and Kocan, 2006; Silva *et al.*, 2009; Hanifah *et al.*, 2011; Madzimure *et al.*, 2011; Merino *et al.*, 2011; Ghosh *et al.*, 2011, 2013).

Vaccines are considered as one of the greatest advances in science with a substantial impact on improving human and animal health. In the early 1990s, vaccines inducing immunological protection to vertebrate hosts against tick infestations were developed and commercialized. The commercial vaccines, Gavac™ (Latin American countries) and TickGARD™ (Australia), contained the recombinant *R. microplus* midgut membrane-bound antigen (BM86) expressed in *Pichia pastoris* and *Escherichia coli*, respectively. The main purpose of these vaccines is to reduce the tick populations and prevalence of tick borne diseases by affecting attachment, feeding, reproduction and development of ticks while they feed on immunized animals and ingesting the blood meal containing antigen specific antibodies that interact with the gut protein and make it non-functional. After ten years of introduction, the vaccine efficacy was assessed and reported positively as a component of IPM programme (de la Fuente, 2007). However, due to wide variations in the vaccine efficacy against different strains of homologous species and very limited efficacy against heterologous species, the overall impact of the TickGARD™/Gavac™ vaccine in animal production system has not been suitably appreciated worldwide.

As multi-tick infestations are the major issues in most of the countries having high animal resources, a universal anti-tick vaccine that renders protection against multiple species of ticks is the commercial need and the steep challenge before the scientific community working on tick vaccines. But the major constrains for the development of improved or universal anti-tick vaccine is identification of antigen (s), which are accessible to the host immune system and capable of imparting protection to both homologous and heterologous species. Along with the identification of vaccine candidates, other key factors *viz.*

a) Adjuvant - Vaccine formulation,

b) Vaccine doses

c) Vaccination interval and frequency

d) Route of administration and

e) Host genetic factors also play a major role in developing successful vaccination.

The identification of genes which are conserved across the different species of ticks and the molecules essential for both tick survival and pathogen transmission are likely to contribute to the discovery of novel vaccine strategies for the simultaneous control of ticks and tick-borne pathogens (de la Fuente *et al.*, 2006, 2007). Moreover, the finding of antigenic protein (s) which are conserved between insects and arachnids and also in different stages of economically important arthropods species may boost the prospects of a pan-arthopod vaccine development (Canales *et al.*, 2009; Prudencio *et al.*, 2010).

The successful development of anti-tick vaccine is complicated, time consuming and challenging. For those involved in the development of vaccines for the control of tick infestations and TBDs, these limitations constitute a challenge that has been approached by developing new platforms for the identification and characterization of candidate tick-derived and pathogen-derived protective antigens. Recent advancement in integration of 'omics' technologies such as immunogenomics, meta-transcriptomics and meta-proteomics with system biology and bioinformatics will help in development of next generation vaccines (Contreras M *et al.*, 2016). Addition to this, advancement in *in-silico* analysis in reverse vaccinology techniques *viz.*, EST library, CattleTickBase, microarrays, sequencing and assembling the tick genomes using new DNA sequencing technologies, in vivo mouse experiments and in-vivo cattle trials may fulfill the field requirements (Lew-Tabor *et al.*, 2010; Maritz-Olivier *et al.*, 2012; Guerrero *et al.*, 2012, 2014; Lew-Tabor and Valle, 2016).

Apart from the research on vaccine candidate search, several factors need to be considered while designing effective vaccines for control of TTBDs (Figure 17.1). For example, tick borne pathogens (TBPs) transmitted through multiple host, it is necessary to consider multiple host for vaccination in that geographic location especially countries like India. It was proved through conducting vaccine trail using aquaporin antigens, where the immune response to aquaporin antigen was differ between hosts.

Adjuvant

An immunologic adjuvant is nothing but any substance that accelerates, prolong, or enhance antigen-specific immune responses when used in combination with specific vaccine antigens. Generally in tick vaccinology, adjuvants are often used to modify or augment the effects of a vaccine candidate by stimulating the immune system. Adjuvants can enhance immunogenicity mainly through two mechanisms: (A) antigen depot formation to ensure slow release and induction of cell-mediated immune responses which are a key precursor in stimulating a strong humoral immune response, (B) inert delivery of antigen to the target immune cells and some adjuvant could confer a dual

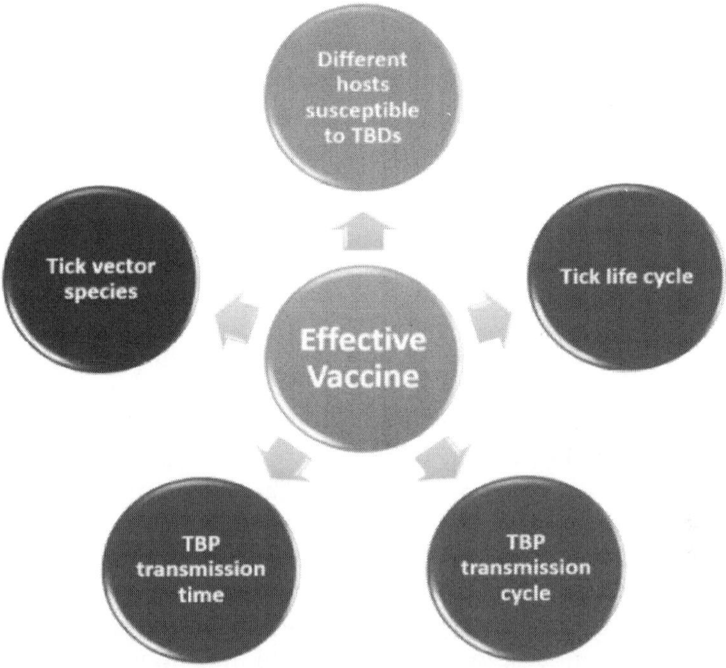

Figure 17.1: Considerable Factors for Designing Effective Vaccines.

function (Ndawula, 2021). Adjuvants accomplish this task by mimicking specific sets of evolutionarily conserved molecules, so called pathogen-associated molecular patterns, which include liposomes, lipopolysaccharide, molecular cages for antigens, components of bacterial cell walls, and endocytosed nucleic acids *etc.* Further, adjuvants may improve stability and prevent degradation of the antigen. Although advances have been made in adjuvant development, a few emulsion-based adjuvants, namely Complete Freund's adjuvant (CFA), Incomplete Freund's adjuvant (FIA), and montanides have been exploited in the formulation of anti-tick vaccines, which act through depot formation at the injection site and slow antigen release to stimulate the immune system. The selection of adjuvants for the formulation of anti-tick vaccines should be based on the adjuvant potency and the minimal induction of side effects. Jackson and Opdebeeck, (1995) compared three adjuvant namely Quil A, Freund's incomplete adjuvant (FIA) and aluminium hydroxide (A1(OH)3) with soluble and membrane midgut antigens of *R. microplus* in sheep and cattle models. Significant antibody levels to midgut membrane antigen (GM) were not detected in the sera of sheep immunized with GM plus A1(OH)3. However, membrane and soluble midgut antigens combined with Quil A generated significantly higher levels of antibodies in sheep than these antigens emulsified in FIA. Similaraly in cattle, soluble midgut antigen (GS) plus Quil A induced significantly higher levels of antibodies compared with GS in FIA. It was concluded that, Quil A was superior to FIA and A1(OH)3 as an adjuvant for these tick antigens. Hence, research work and reports on comparison studies regarding the effect of adjuvants like mineral compounds (*e.g.*, alum, calcium salts), liposomes, bacterial products (*e.g.*, bacterial derived toxins and non-toxins), ISCOMs, tensoactive compounds (*e.g.*, Quil-A), and nanoparticles along with the antigens is essential to prevent the paucity of commercial anti-tick vaccines.

Vaccine Dose Administration

The optimum inoculation dose could vary depending on number of factors like (A) the type of antigen and its ability to trigger different components of immune system, (B) the adjuvant used in the vaccine formulation, whereby each adjuvant has unique characteristics and action mechanisms, (C) route of administration, and (D) host related factors. Generally, there is a consensus that the antigen dose impacts proportionally on humoral immune responses and the vaccine protection outcome. However, when primed with a high antigen dose, the antibody titer levels off earlier and the antibody formation mechanism will be impaired after immunization. Ultimately, inoculating a high antigen concentration also induces vaccine immune-tolerance, which in return reduces vaccine efficacy. In principle, an equal vaccine dose should be administered irrespective of the size, body weight or breed. Since the vaccine dose depends on the number of circulating lymphoid molecules. Inoculating a vaccine dose based on animal body weight could lead to undesirable immunological effects, which in tuns leads to reduction in vaccine efficacy. Therefore, to accurately determine the optimum anti-tick vaccine dose, researchers should exploit the humoral immune response kinetics curve by performing immunological studies with a wide range of antigen concentrations. Alternatively, the prime vaccine dose may be determined based on existing information about similar antigens.

Booster Vaccine Dose

The aim of boost vaccination is to elicit a specific, robust, and long-lasting immune protection. Although booster vaccination follows the earlier-described action mechanism, the immune response is faster. Since, the booster vaccine exploits the prime vaccine-induced memory B cells which change into plasma B cells to produce antigen-specific antibodies. Hanna and Peters (1971) illustrated that priming an animal with a low vaccine dose leads to a stronger secondary immune response than priming with a higher vaccine dose. However, until now the optimum anti-tick vaccine prime dose is not known. Hence, research on the effect of administration of a high booster vaccine dose linked with the avidity of the secondary antibodies and administering half the prime vaccine dose as a booster vaccine dose for stronger humoral response is need to be studied.

Vaccination Interval and Frequency

Vaccine efficacy depends on the ability of the memory B cells to generate effective antibodies after inoculation with the cognate antigen. In humans, when there is continuous immune system exposure to the cognate antigen that was used for priming, the protection can last for decades (Ahamd and Gray, 1996). Similar phenomenon could occur with anti-tick vaccines, particularly with non-concealed antigens or concealed/non-concealed (those expressed in saliva and other tissues) (Hassan *et al.*, 2020). However, the response could be slower considering that a minute quantity of salivary proteins is inoculated during tick feeding and the half-life of serum immunoglobulins is very short (1–3 weeks) (Viera *et al.*, 1986, 1988). Therefore, to sustain the immune response, it is necessary to inoculate booster vaccine dose(s) by taking into account of vaccination booster frequency and number of doses to maintain immune response. Evidence shows that booster vaccination at a short interval after the priming does not lead to induction of a stronger secondary immune response; rather it interferes with the primary response, which leads to immune tolerance. Hence, researchers should consider the humoral immune-response kinetics curve while determining the interval for administering the booster doses. In humans, the humoral immune-response self-termination feedback mechanism occurs at least 2–3 months after the primary vaccination, which is optimal to induce a robust secondary adaptive immune response. Often the booster anti-tick vaccine doses are administered after two weeks. This suggests that most of the anti-tick vaccines are administered before the prime immune response has waned which could affect the immune memory induction, and hence the vaccine protection efficacy. Vaccination of cattle with Bm86 (Gavacplus) against *R. microplus*, demonstrated that one booster dose per year was sufficient to maintain humoral protection and that the booster dose should not be administered until the antibody titer drops below 1: 640 (Vagas *et al.*, 2010). Therefore, it is also possible that anti-tick vaccines, particularly those derived from proteins expressed in the tick saliva and other tissues, may induce a longer protection.

Route of Vaccination

Human vaccines are commonly administered via the parenteral intra-muscular (IM) route. Generally, vaccination via the IM route induces higher and quicker adaptive immune responses since they drain directly into the lymphatic system in comparison to than vaccination via the other dermal routes. In addition, IM vaccine inoculation induces fewer adverse effects than the dermal route (Wahl *et al.*, 1987). To enhance the anti-tick vaccine immune protection, researchers may consider using the IM route for prime dose inoculation and other dermal routes for booster dose inoculation. For instance, McCluskie *et al.* (2002) illustrate that parenteral prime mucosal boost vaccination elicits a diverse immune responses. It is worthwhile to further exploit the benefits conferred by adjuvants when combined with vaccines since the route of vaccination is influenced by type of adjuvants (Gupta *et al.*, 2015, Uddowla *et al.*, 2007).

Approach of Assessing Vaccine Efficacy

In general, the current approach of assessing the efficacy of tick vaccines is based on one-host tick species. This entails determining the relative weight reduction of engorged female ticks, eggs, and viable larvae from vaccinated and non-vaccinated hosts. In Indian condition, multi-tick infestation is more problematic, since ticks prefers multi-host for feeding activity Hence, it is not possible to extensively assess the anti-tick vaccine efficacy and effectiveness using the current approach. Therefore, to develop effective universal anti-tick vaccines, there is need for incorporation of few factors as listed for assessing population reduction and mortality of single- and multiple-host ticks *viz.*,

1. Assess the humeral immune response kinetics,
2. Assess adult tick engorgement (vaccine effect on the feeding of female ticks).
3. Vaccine effect on adult tick egg laying (oviposition).
4. Vaccine effect on egg hatchability.
5. Vaccine effect on larval feeding.
6. Vaccine effect on larval molting.
7. Vaccine effect on nymph feeding.

The vaccine overall efficacy is a product of the vaccine relative effect on different key biological parameters (*e.g.*, tick feeding, egg laying, egg hatching, larvae and nymph molting) among ticks from the vaccinated (Vac) and control (Cont) group. The parameters are: TF (Tick feeding), TE (egg laying), TH (egg hatchability), TL (larvae feeding), and TN (nymph feeding). Therefore, percentage overall efficacy (E per cent): E per cent = 100 × [1–[[TFvac/TFcont] × [TEcont/TEvac] × [THcont/THvac] × [TLcont/TLvac] × [TNcont/TNvac]

= 100 × [1 – [ETF × ETE × ETH × ETL × ETN]]

The rationale is that these are the visible indicators/markers of tick population growth under field conditions (Cunha *et al.*, 2013, Aguirre *et al.*, 2015).

Assessing Vaccine Efficacy Including Pathogen Effect

Recently, De la fuente*et al* (2017) proposed a risk assessment model for tick borne diseases which was earlier developed by Kilpatrick *et al.* (2005) for mosquito-borne West Nile virus. Accordingly, TBDs risk will be estimated as, Risk (R) = A x Fmx P x Cv x T x S, where A is the diversity of the tick species in the study area, Fm is the fraction of blood meals taken from natural hosts for TBP, P is the TBP infection prevalence in the tick vector species, Cv is an index of tick vector competence corresponding to the fraction of TBP-infected ticks that will transmit pathogen after bite, T is the attachment success and feeding time of a tick vector species, and S is the vertebrate host (human, companion, farm or wild animal) susceptibility to TBP (de la fuente*et al.*, 2017). Considering the risk assessment of the TBDs, the efficacy (E) of a vaccine to decrease the risk for TTBDs can be estimated as E = E1 x E2 x E3 x E4 x E5 (Table 17.1).

Table 17.1: Efficacy of Vaccine Assessment Formulae in Relation to Risk Factors

Component	*Represents*	*Related to risk assessment*
E1	A and Fm	Reduction in ticks number includes, feeding, oviposition and fertility. Reduction in tick number to be calculated for single host and multiple-host ticks as discussed in de la fuente and Contreras, 2015 and Aguirre *et al.*, 2015, respectively.
E2	P	Reduction in TBP infection and multiplication in the tick vector
E3	Cv	Reduction in TBP transmission by the tick vector
E4	T	Reduction in tick attachment and feeding time
E5	S	Reduction in host pathogen infection

Based on this model, research strategies should be implemented to control TTBDs. For examples, ticks involved in transmission of viruses, vaccine molecules to be identified with more emphasis on affecting tick attachment and feeding time (E4), and/or reduction in host TBP infection (E5) to protect hosts from these TBDs. In case of most bacterial and protozoan pathogens, tick borne pathogen transmission time after tick bite is important factor since, they require several hours of tick feeding on host for transmission in comparison to viruses. Henceforth, blocking the pathogen transmission is much easier compare to tick borne viruses in host vaccinated with candidates affecting tick infestations (E1) and TBP infection and multiplication in the tick vector (E2). Besides, tick and tick borne diseases need to be addressed through novel tools with promising potential in arthropod vector control (Benelli, 2018).

Overall, all the questions outlined above need to be addressed through research efforts from public health experts, epidemiologists, parasitologists, biologists and epidemiologists. However, more efficient health system infrastructures and entomological capacity are urgently required in endemic countries to ensure an effective management of vectors. In India, Entomology laboratory, ICAR-IVRI is solely working on tick vaccines. Hence, there is an urgent need of trained manpower in tick research to explore the immunological related factors that influence vaccine and identification of new vaccine candidates.

Chapter 18

Role of Semiochemicals in the Control of Arthropods

Suman Kumar, G. Das, Rupesh Verma, S. Nath, Supriya Sachan, Ravi Kumar Khare and Vikram Punia

*Department of Veterinary Parasitology,
College of Veterinary Science and A.H., NDVSU,
Jabalpur – 482001, Madhya Pradesh*

Introduction

Arthropods of veterinary importance parasitize our livestock and are responsible for economic losses to farmers and livestock industry. The current control strategy is mainly based on the use of chemical insecticides. But due to indiscriminate uses of chemical insecticides, many arthropods have started developing resistance against these chemicals. Development of insecticidal resistance led the search of alternative strategies for arthropod control and one of those strategies is to use of semiochemicals. Semiochemicals are bioactive compounds which are responsible to convey specific messages by modifying the physiological behaviours in individuals of either same species or other species (Sonenshine 2004). Since the identification, semiochemicals are regarded as one of the tools in arthropod control strategies (Karlson and Luscher 1959).

Classification of Semiochemicals

A. Allelochemicals

These are bioactive compounds, produced and emitted by individuals of one species that bring the behavioural changes in individual of other species (Tewari *et al.*, 2014).

a. **Allomones:** Allomones are bioactive compounds, produced and emitted by individuals of a species and bring the behavioural changes in individual of a different species that benefit the emitting individuals.

b. **Kairomones:** These compounds are produced and emitted by one species and detected by another species, which enables them to locate or identify the host species, food, *etc.*, and get benefited.

c. **Synomones:** Synomones are produced by individuals of one species provoke a response beneficial to both the emitter and the receiver (Sonenshine 2006).

d. **Apneumones:** Apneumones are substances produced by non-living materials that elicit behavioural changes which is beneficial to the receiving organism but harmful to a second organism in the non-living material.

B. Pheromones

These are the chemicals produced by an individual that bring the changes in individual's behaviour of the same species. Pheromones are of two types, primer pheromones and releaser pheromones. Release pheromones may be sub-divided into the following types:

a. **Aggregation pheromones**: These bioactive compounds are produced by one or both sexes for bringing both sexes in the proximity of each other together for feeding and reproduction (Tinzaara *et al.*, 2002).

b. **Attraction-Aggregation-Attachment-pheromones:** The attraction–aggregation–attachment pheromones are a mix of organic volatiles secreted by the feeding adult males of the genus *Amblyomma* which are capable of attracting non-feeding con-specific nymphs and adults of either sex to form feeding clusters on bovine or other hosts (Sonenshine 2004).

c. **Arrestment Pheromones**: These are non-volatile compounds and recognized by ticks when they come in direct contact with them, and their activities start getting ceased. These compounds are species-specific and active against unfed immature stages as well as the adult.

d. **Alarm pheromones:** Alarm pheromones are anti-predator chemicals that warn the individuals of the same species about the presence or absence of an enemy.

e. **Oviposition-deterrent:** These compounds assist females of some insect species to prevent egg deposition on the hosts, which have previously been utilized by con-specifics, so a reduction in the intra-specific competition (Stelinski *et al.*, 2007).

f. **Sex pheromones:** Sex pheromones are generally emitted by individuals of one sex that attract individuals of the opposite sex for mating. Some of the sex pheromones of insects are effectively used in the integrated pest management (IPM) system in agriculture (Nandagopal *et al.*, 2008).

g. **Attractant Sex Pheromone:** Attractant sex pheromone (2, 6-dichlorophenol) is produced by Metastriate tick, which is responsible for initiating the mate-finding activity in some hard ticks. Recognizing this pheromone, fully fed or feeding males get excited and start crawling in search of the females emitting pheromone.

h. **Mounting Sex Pheromone:** Mounting sex pheromone is a contact sex pheromone produced by females, which enables males to spot suitable mating partners (Ranju *et al.*, 2012). Mounting occurs only if the males perceive the mounting sex pheromones. In hard ticks, cholesteryl esters are recognized as components of mounting sex pheromone (Sonenshine 2006).

i. **Genital Sex Pheromones**: These are pheromones found in few closely related tick species, wood tick and *D. andersoni*, in which ecdysteroids are found to be an essential component of their genital sex pheromone. The male ticks detect the genital sex pheromone with the help of their chelicerae.

j. **Trail pheromones:** The trail pheromones are useful in finding mates or using food resources more effectively. In the case of social or migrating insects, these pheromones help in maintaining the cohesion and social integration of the colony (McPheron *et al.*, 1997).

h. **Royal pheromones:** These pheromones are used by the queens (and by kings in the case of termites). Royal pheromones let workers recognize the queen/king and care for them apart from maintaining the reproductive division of labour (Funaro *et al.*, 2018).

Control Strategies based Semiochemicals

a. **Detection and Monitoring:** Insect sex pheromones are used for attracting insects and catching them in the traps. The captured insects in the traps indicate whether a particular insect is present in a given geographical area and also the time of its seasonal flight period. Detection and monitoring is a simple and most commonly used strategy for determining the time for insecticide use (Wall *et al.*, 1987).

b. **Mass trapping:** In this technique the semiochemicals which are involved in mate finding and bringing behavioural changes, such as aggregation pheromones, sex pheromones *etc.* are used to attract and trap the targeted insects. Keeping records of mass trapping of a given area is very important in formulating effective control strategies against the particular insect group (Cork *et al.*, 2003).

c. **Lucitrap:** Lucitrap is a device developed for the control of sheep blowflies. It comprises attractants such as sodium sulfide and a mixture of butanoic acid, 2-mercaptoethanol, and indole in a dispenser and a 2-part plastic trap which helps in for catching and holding the trapped flies (Urech *et al.*, 2004).

d. **Adult mosquito traps**: The devices developed for adult mosquitoes are BG-Sentinel trap and CDC-Autocidal Gravid Ovitrap. The gravid traps are user-friendly in comparison to BG-Sentinel traps. The traps release ammonia, fatty acid and lactic acid as attractant.

e. **Mating disruption:** In the last few decades, mating disruption method was the most useful approach in the insect control programme. It involves the use of synthetic pheromones to mimic the species-specific female sex pheromone in a limited area that prevents male insects from finding mates. Introducing the sex pheromone into the habitat reduces the chances of males finding their mate for successful mating. Resulting, the subsequent population reduces, and fewer larvae are present to cause damage (Witzgall *et al.*, 2010; Mafra-Neto *et al.*, 2014).

f. **Tick lure and kill strategies:** Use of pheromone alone sometimes may not be useful; so the combination of attractants and acaricides along with a sustained-release technology has been tested against the ticks.

Two devices incorporated with 2, 6-dichlorophenol and acaricides have been tested against the ticks. The first one is incorporated with 2, 6-dichlorophenol and propoxur along with oily substance against *D. variabilis* (Sonenshine *et al.*, 1985). The second delivery device is tick decoy. The tick decoy was developed to attract *D. variabilis* males to a bead-shaped plastic spherule (female mimic) using 2, 6-dichlorophenol, cholesteryl oleate along with propoxur.

Conclusion

Semiochemicals have been used in several ways in the arthropods control as they are considered as safer and environment-friendly due to their low persistency. The main hurdles in use of these compounds are their volatility and lack of stability. Therefore, sustained-released formulations could be the key in enhancing the semiochemicals activity by slowing down their degradation. Researches on semiochemicals in arthropods control should be intended in the development of the formulations of technologies for their sustained-release, and enhancing trapping efficiency.

REFERENCES

Allan SA, Sonenshine DE (2002) Evidence of an assembly pheromone in the black-legged deer tick, *Ixodes scapularis*. J Chem Ecol 28: 15-27

Berger RS (1972) 2, 6-Dichilorophenol, sex pheromone of the lone star tick. Science. 177: 704-705

Broce AB. (1988). An improved Alsynite trap for stable flies, *Stomoxys calcitrans* (Diptera: Muscidae). J Med Entomol 25: 406-409

Cork A, Alam SN, Rouf FM, Talekar NS (2003). Female sex pheromone of brinjal fruit and shoot borer, *Leucinodes orbonalis* (Lepidoptera: Pyralidae): trap optimization and application in IPM trials. Bull Entomol Res 93: 107-113

Funaro CF, Böröczky K, Vargo EL, Schal C (2018). Identification of a queen and king recognition pheromone in the subterranean termite *Reticulitermes flavipes*. Proc Nat Acad Sci 15: 3888-893

Karlson P Luscher M (1959). Pheromones: a new term for a class of biologically active substances. Nature 183: 55–56

Mafra-Neto A, Fettig CJ, Unson AS, Rodriguez-Saona C *et al.* (2014) Development of specialized pheromone and lure application technologies (SPLAT®) for management of Coleopteran pests in agricultural and forest systems. Biopesticides: State of the art and future opportunities. American Chemical Society pp 211- 242

McPheron LJ, Seybold SJ, Storer AJ, Wood DL *et al.* (1997) Effects of enantiomeric blend of verbenone on response of Ifps paraconfusus to naturally produced aggregation pheromone in the laboratory. J Chem Ecol 23: 2825–2839

Nandagopal V, Prakash A, Rao J (2008). Know the pheromones: Basics and its application. J Biopest 1: 210-215

Njiru BN, Mukabana WR, Takken W, Knols BG (2006) Trapping of the malaria vector *Anopheles gambiae* with odour-baited MM-X traps in semi-field conditions in western Kenya. Malar J 5: 39-47

Snyder D, Cernicchiaro N, Allan SA, Cohnstaedt LW (2016) Insecticidal sugar baits for adult biting midges. Med Vet Entomol 30: 209-217

Sonenshine DE (2004) Pheromones and other semiochemicals of ticks and their use in tick control. Parasitol 129: 405-425

Sonenshine DE (2006) Tick pheromones and their use in tick control. Ann Rev Entomol 51: 557- 580

Sonenshine DE (2017) Pheromones: Function and use in insect and tick control. Old Dominion University, Norfolk, VA, United States pp. 1-53.

Sonenshine DE, Taylor D, Corrigan G (1985) Studies to evaluate the effectiveness of sex pheromone-impregnated formulations for control of populations of the American dog tick, *Dermacentor variabilis* (Say) (Acari: Ixodidae). Exp Appl Acarol. 1: 23-34

Stelinski LL, Oakleaf R, Rodriguez-Saona C (2007) Oviposition-deterring pheromone deposited on blueberry fruit by the parasitic wasp, *Diachasma alloeum*. Behaviour 144: 429-446

Suckling DM (2015) Can we replace toxicants, achieve biosecurity, and generate market position with semiochemicals?. Front Ecol Evol 3: 17-24

Tinzaara W, Dicke M, van Huis A, Gold CS (2002) Use of infochemicals in pest management with special reference to the banana weevil, Cosmopolites sordidus (Germar) (Coleoptera: Curculionidae). Int J Trop Insect Sc 22 : 241-261

Urech R, Green PE, Rice MJ, Brown GW, *et al.* (2004). Composition of chemical attractants affects trap catches of the Australian sheep blowfly, *Lucilia cuprina,* and other blowflies. J Chem Ecol 30: 851-866

Wall, C, Garthwaite DG, Blood Smyth JA, Sherwood A (1987). The efficacy of sex-attractant monitoring for the pea moth, *Cydia nigricana,* in England, 1980–1985. Ann appl Biol 110: 223–229

Witzgall P, Kirsch P, Cork A (2010) Sex pheromones and their impact on pest management. J Chem Ecol 36: 80-100.

Chapter 19

Genetic Control of Screwworm Fly and Mosquito

P. Azhahianambi

Translational Research Platform for Veterinary Biologicals, Centre for Animal Health Studies, Tamil Nadu Veterinary and Animal Sciences University, Madhavaram, Chennai, Tamil Nadu

Introduction

Alternatives to chemical-based insect control are the need of the hour for sustainable livestock production to ensure food security in future. Selection of insecticide resistant insect population, environmental impact of insecticides, insecticide residues, organic livestock products market expansion and non-availability of new generation insecticides in near future are the key issues which compel the scientists to look for sustainable alternative approaches to control insect population. Among the various sustainable insect control methods, genetic control of insects is an insect population control method with promising outlook. Sterile Insect Technique (SIT), Genetically modified (GM) insects and Incompatible Insect Release (IIT), are the three important genetic methods which have the potential to suppress/eradicate an insect population in a wider geographical area such as a state or country. Genetic control of insects is an essential technology which would help the human race to win over the multi-insecticide resistant insect population, if any arise in future. In the same way, this technology would also help to stop the spread of deadly vector borne diseases. SIT is based on radiation of pupal stages of target insect species and it has been useful in eradicating an important livestock pest New World Screwworm (NWS) in America. GM insects for genetic control purpose are made by inserting lethal genes into the target insect genome through transgenic insect technology with and without gene drive. IIT is a para-genetic approach which is based on mating incompatibility between the mass-released *Wolbachia* transfected male and un-infected wild female insects. The success stories on eradication of screwworm from north and central America using SIT and suppression of *Aedes aegypti* mosquito population in Brazil using GM mosquitoes (*Aedes aegypti* OX5034) are really encouraging in nature.

Applications of Insect Genetic Control Methods

- ☆ Population control of target insects (Suppress insect population)
- ☆ Eradication of an insect population from a geographical area
- ☆ Control of vector borne diseases (*e.g.*, Control of *Anopheles* mosquito to control malaria)
- ☆ Insect population eradication/suppression in a wider geographical area

1. Sterile Insect Technique (SIT)

SIT works by releasing mass-reared, radiation-treated sterile insects of a target species. The sterile males compete with the wild males for female insects for mating. If a wild female mates with a sterile male, the wild female insect cannot produce viable offspring, thus reducing the next generation's insect population. Repeated release of sterile insects can eventually reduce the wild insect population to very low levels or zero and hence reduce the damage or spread of disease. This technique relies on the rearing of the target insect in large numbers in specialized production centres, sterilization with ionizing radiation such as X-ray and gamma ray and sustained sequential release of the sterilized insects over a selected target area. Insects subjected to specific dose of ionizing radiation would become sterile due to "chromosome translocation" and "dicentric chromosomes".

e.g., Eradication of New World Screwworm in North and Central America using SIT

Disadvantages of SIT

- ☆ Cannot be applied in all insect species. Some insect species require very high dose of radiation to achieve the sterility that could compromise with their mating and survival fitness
- ☆ Require expensive infrastructure
- ☆ Radiation hazard
- ☆ Population density dependent growth and emergence in mosquitoes
- ☆ Repeated mating behavior of insect species. New world Screwworm (NWS) female flies resist the second mating and that is one of the main reasons behind the success of the SIT

- ✰ Male and female fly separation is not possible
- ✰ Invasion of gravid female insects from other zone or nearby countries

2. Genetically Modified (GM) Insects

GM insects are transgenic insects carrying foreign gene in their genome which is heritable. GM insects are created by inserting an effect or gene into their genome to render the GM insects either with bi-sexual lethal or female lethal phenotype. The gene insertion in the germ-line of insects is done through transgenic insect technology. There are three types of GM insects carrying dominant lethal genes being used in the population control of insects *viz.* i) **Transgenic Sexing Strains** (TSS) ii) **Bi-sex RIDL** (Bi-sex-Release of Insects with Dominant Lethal gene) and iii) **fsRIDL** (Female Specific-Release of Insects with Dominant Lethal gene).

TSS-GM insects are "Male only" insects created for the application in the SIT, where segregation of male and female insects is not possible. TSS-GM insects carry lethal gene expressed only in female insects and "male only" colony is reared in the laboratory under specific diet conditions. As the lethal gene is under the control of Tetracycline operator (Tet-Off), the breeding colony is reared with tetracycline and the male only colony is reared without tetracycline. The insect colony reared without tetracycline would have only male insects. The male pupae would undergo ionizing radiation and subsequently be released into the nature. This strategy avoids the release of radiated female insects into nature and improves the efficiency of SIT. Further, this would reduce the use of ionizing radiation as the male pupa needs comparatively less radiation dose.

RIDL technology which is an alternate method to SIT where transgenic insects carrying dominant lethal gene specifically expressed in female insects (fsRIDL)or dominant lethal genes expressed in both male and female insects (Bi-sex RIDL) can be used to suppress/eradicate the target insect population. The main advantage of this method is no need to use ionizing radiation and affordable (**Figures 19.1 and 19.2**).

Sex Specific Expression of Lethal Genes

Somatic sex determination occurs in fruit fly by alternate RNA splicing of transformer gene (*tra*) and double sex gene (*dsx*). This sex specific alternate RNA splicing mechanism in insects is being exploited to express the lethal gene only in females and ultimately to control insect population. The commonly used lethal genes are **tetracycline transactivator** (*tTa*) and pro-apoptotic (*hid-* ***Head Involution Defective)*** gene. The lethality of *tTa* is thought to be due to *"transcriptional squelching"*, a biological phenomenon in whicha transcriptional activator acts to inhibit the expression of another gene. High levels of expression of the *tTA* transcription factor are thought to be toxic to insects due to either transcriptional squelching or interference with protein ubiquitination. GM male insects carrying dominant lethal gene (lethal gene is not expressed in male insects) released into nature would mate with wild females and the resulting female progenies would die. Eradication or population suppression of insects can be attained by multiple and programmed release of transgenic male insects carrying dominant lethal gene.

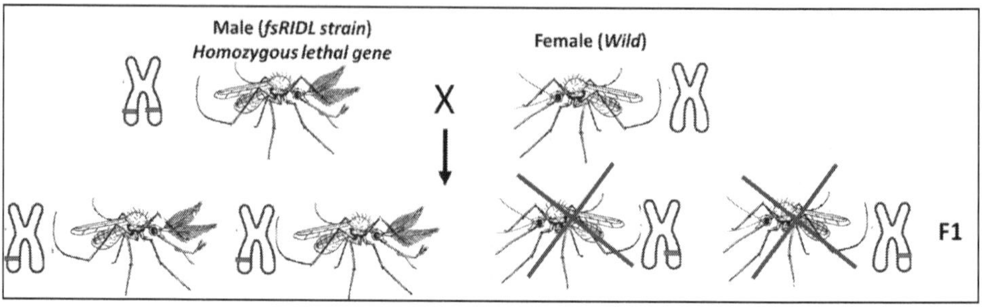

Figure 19.1: Female Lethal Phenotype.

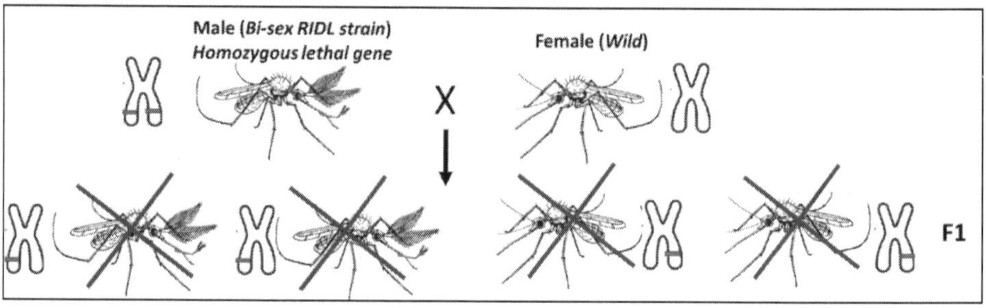

Figure 19.2: Bi-sex Lethal Phenotype.

Limitations of GM Insect Technology

- ☆ Genetically Modified organism tag (Socio-political issue)
- ☆ Horizontal Gene Transfer or Lateral gene transfer (Movement of *genetic* material other than vertical transmission)
- ☆ Mating with related insect species
- ☆ GM insect technology is not available for all the insect species
- ☆ Eradication of an insect species (Ethical issue)
- ☆ Unforeseen consequences
- ☆ Limited commercial potential

3. Incompatible Insect Release (IIT)

This approach works by releasing mass-reared, *Wolbachia* transfected male insects. The *Wolbachia* transfected males compete with the wild males for mating with wild female insects. If a *Wolbachia* free wild female mates with a *Wolbachia* transfected male, then it will have no viable offspring, thus reducing the next generation's population. Repeated release of *Wolbachia* transfected male insects can eventually reduce the target insect population to very low levels or zero. The male and female insect species are transfected with *Wolbachia* and mass reared in a laboratory facility. The *Wolbachia* transfected male pupae (smaller pupal size) are physically segregated, mass reared and released. The mating incompatibility of *Wolbachia*-male and wild female insect is due to "*cytoplasmic incompatibility*" phenomenon which leads to loss of mitotic synchrony and early embryonic death. Mating incompatibility also exists between different *Wolbachia* strains infected insects (*Wolbachia* strain A and *Wolbachia* B strain infected insects) (**Figures 19.3 and 19.4**)

e.g., *Wolbachia* is absent in *Aedes aegypti* and *Anopheles* mosquitoes. *Wolbachia*-*Aedes* mosquitoes reduced *A. aegypti* mosquito populations in Singapore towns by up to 98 per cent (Project *Wolbachia* Singapore)

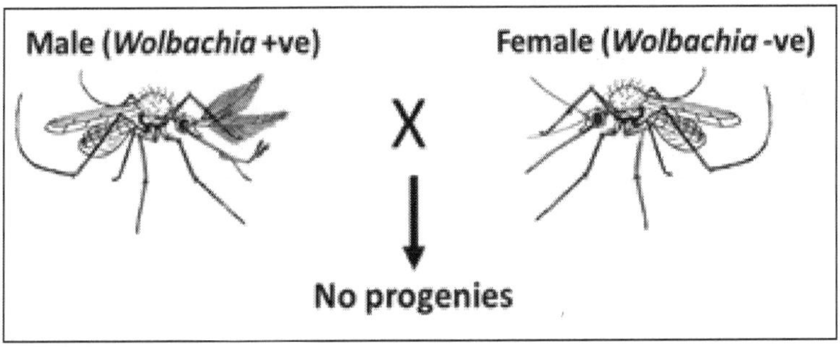

Figure 19.3: Uni-directional CI.

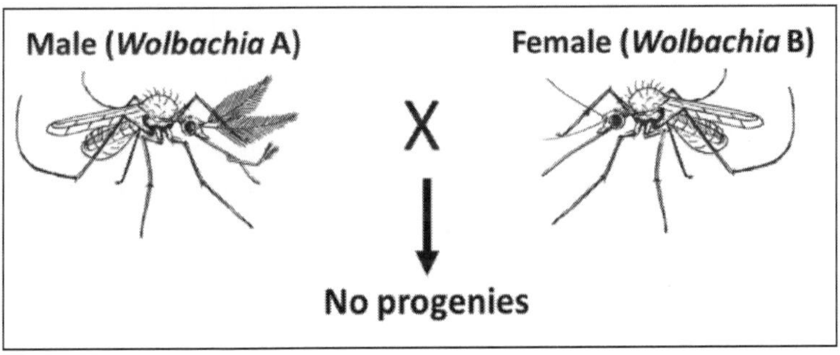

Figure 19.4: Bi-directional CI.

Disadvantages

- ☆ Poor understanding of CI mechanism and different *Wolbachia* strains
- ☆ Not useful in all insect species (*e.g.*, No vertical transmission in *Anopheles gambiae*)
- ☆ Unknown status of *Wolbachia* infected insect population in an area

- ☆ *Wolbachia* transfected male insects can produce viable eggs with Wild *Wolbachia* infected female insects.
- ☆ Repeated mating behavior of the insects
- ☆ Can be used only in insects that allow the establishment of *Wolbachia* in their reproductive organs.

4. The Art and Science of Creation of GM Insects

GM insect technology is a molecular biology technique designed to deliver transgenes into the germline of insects with stable transformation which is heritable. The vectors used in the stable germline transformation of insects are transposable elements (*e.g., piggyBac*), CRISPR/Cas9 or Homing Endonucleases (I-SceI). Transposable elements used to transform the insects are DNA transposons which mobilize inside the insect genome by cut and paste mechanism. *piggyBac* is the commonly used DNA transposable element in the creation of GM insects. *piggyBac* transposon vector loaded with dominant lethal genes is introduced into the genome of target insect species to create a transgenic insect line with female lethal (fsRIDL) or bi-sex lethal (Bi-sex RIDL) phenotype. This can be achieved by transforming the germline of the insect embryos by microinjection of the transposable elements carrying lethal gene and marker gene. In case of fsRIDL, female sex specific splicing intron DNA sequences are placed in between the promoter sequence and lethal gene in such a way to express the lethal genes only female insects and not in male insects. The expression of lethal genes in GM insects can be inhibited by adding tetracycline in the larval and adult diet as the lethal is under the control of Tetracycline Operator sequence (Tet-Off system). Withdrawal of tetracycline in the larval diet leads to death of all female insects and emergence of male only insect population which can be used to release into the nature. Homozygous male insect strains carrying female lethal gene will be released into the nature to competitively mate with wild female insects which in turn would result in progenies of heterozygous genotype carrying female lethal genes. The heterozygous female insects carrying the female lethal genes would die in their early life due to the lack of tetracycline in nature. The heterozygous male population would survive in the nature and competitively mate with wild female insects and spread the lethal genes in to the population.

In CRISPR/Cas9 based insect transgenesis, the Cas9 endonuclease and Single guide RNA (sgRNA) expressed in the insect reproductive organs target the specific PAM sites in the insect genome and make double strand break in the target site. The transformation vector consists of homologous host sequences in the left and right side of the vector, would integrate into the cut site by Homology Directed Repair.

5. How to Create a GM Insect with Female Lethal Phenotype?

I. Isolation and characterization of insect species specific transformer gene (*tra*) and double sex (*dsx*) gene and identification of female specific splicing intron(s)

1. RNA isolation from male and female insects
2. RT-PCR with degenerate primers designed against conserved amino acid blocks by comparing tra/dsx gene sequence of *Drosophila* sp., *Lucilia* sp. and New World Screwworm.
3. 5′ and 3′ RACE-PCR to obtain full length cDNA of tra/dsx gene and DNA sequencing
4. PCR amplification of *tra* gene from insect genomic DNA using exon-specific primers and DNA sequencing
5. Characterization of exons and introns of *tra/dsx* gene of male and female insects and identification of female sex specific splicing intron

IIa. Making of transformation vector and *piggyBac* helper plasmid

Transformation Vector with piggyBac Ends

Marker gene (*e.g.*, GFP) under the transcription control of insect heat shock promoter and lethal gene (*e.g.*, Tetracycline transactivator) under the control of insect minimal heat shock promoter which is downstream to the Tet Operator (*TetO*) sequence. Female specific splicing tra/dsx intron is inserted between lethal gene tTAV and the minimal heat shock promoter. The expression of lethal gene is regulated by *tet-Off* system (No lethal gene expression in the presence of tetracycline) **(Figure 19.5).**

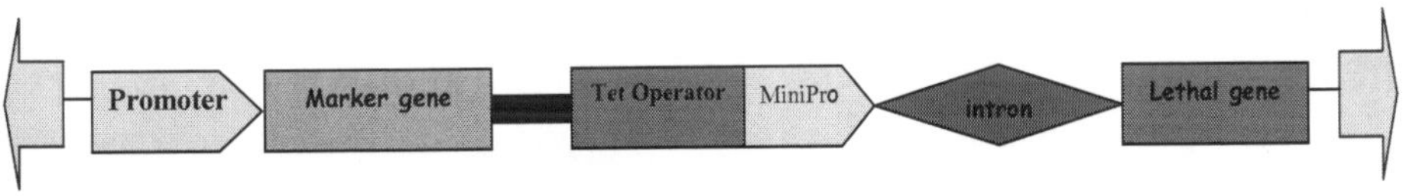

Figure 19.5: *piggyBac* Transformation Vector with Lethal Gene and Female Specific Splicing Intron.

PiggyBac Helper Plasmid

Insect heat shock promoter driving the expression of *piggyBac* transposase. **(Figure 19.6)**

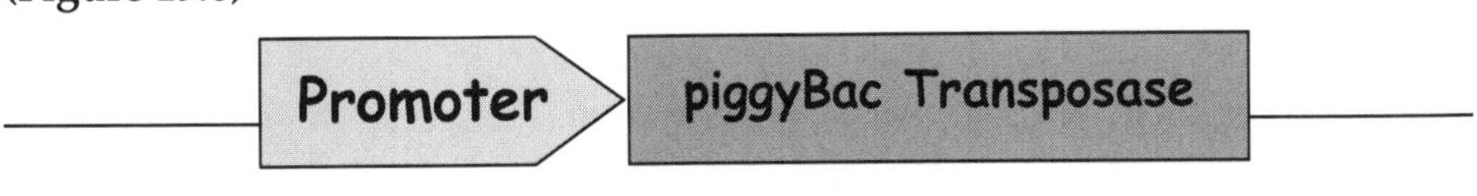

Figure 19.6: *piggyBac* Transposase Expressing Helper Plasmid.

IIb. Making of transformation vector with CRISPR/Cas9 gene editing technology

Transformation Vector Containing Host Homologous Sequences

The transformation vector similar to the afore mentioned design, where the *piggyBac* ends are replaced with insect genome sequences and the entire cassette would be integrated into insect genome by homologous recombination **(Figure 19.7)**

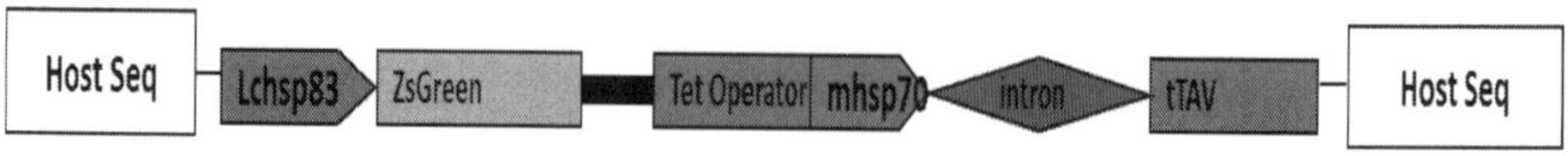

Figure 19.7: Transformation Vector with Flanked by Host DNA Sequence Homologous to each Side of Cas9 Nuclease Cut-Site.

CRISPR/Cas9 Gene Editing Cassette

The cassette consists of Cas9 ORF with a promoter (*nanos* promoter) driving the expression in reproductive organs of insects, and single guide RNA with spacer sequences targeting the insect genomes. The spacer sequences are designed down-stream to the 5′NGG Proto Spacer Adjacent (PAM) sequences of target insect genome to precisely integrate the transformation vector into the target site **(Figure 19.8).**

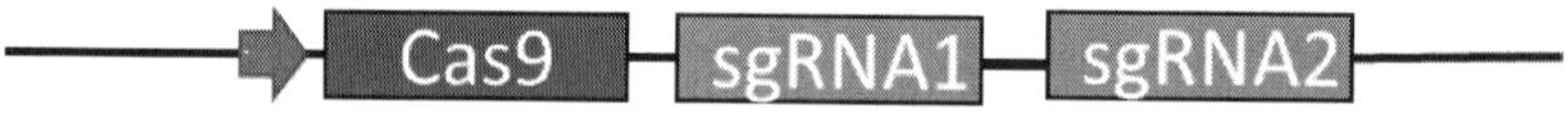

Figure 19.8: Cassette Expressing the Cas9 Endonuclease and Single Guide RNA.

III. Micro-injection of transformation vector plasmid and *piggyBac* helper plasmid into fresh insect embryos or CRISPR/cas9 cassette and transformation vector with host sequences

Transformation vector and helper plasmid DNA at specific concentrations will be used for microinjection. Quartz and silicon glass needles are used to deliver the DNA mixture into the posterior pole of the insect embryos. Inject the embryos one by one at the posterior pole and deposit the DNA into the syncytial germ cells at the posterior pole. Adjust the volume of DNA deposited into the embryo by adjusting the pressure and duration of injection. Few picolitres of DNA delivered at right place inside egg at right time is enough to create a transgenic insect. The larvae hatching out from the microinjected embryos are called **G0** larvae.

IV. Screening and Genetic crosses to obtain homozygous transgenic lines

a) Screening of adult fly for the expression of marker gene

Depending upon the nature of the promoter driving the expression of marker gene, the spatial and temporal expression of marker genes (EGFP, DsRed) can be viewed under specific excitation wavelength of UV light.

b) Genetic crosses to obtain homozygous line

1. Rearing the insects in the presence of tetracycline to prevent the female lethality in the breeding insect population. The expression of lethal gene in female insects can be repressed by feeding them tetracycline containing insect food.
2. Generation 0 (G0) adults will be out-crossed with laboratory colony insects to obtain G1 larvae. G1 larvae will be screened for the expression of marker gene under fluorescent microscope using appropriate filters.
3. G1 transgenic adults will be out crossed with laboratory colony insects to obtain G2 larvae. Screening of G2 larvae and separation of transgenic larvae.
4. Inbreeding of G2 adults and subsequent generation up to G5 to obtain homozygous transgenic lines

V. Characterization of Transgenic Line

piggyBac specific inverse PCR and transposable element display (TE display) will be done to identify the genomic location of the different transgenic lines.

VI. Female Lethal Test

1. Homozygous transgenic insect lines out crossed with laboratory colony insects and the resulting eggs will be placed in medium with and without tetracycline.
2. Calculation emerging adult Male: Female insect sex ratio in the presence and absence of tetracycline
3. Select the homozygous transgenic insect lines showing 100 per cent female lethal phenotype

VII. Laboratory Cage Study/Field Cage Study and Risk Evaluation

The selected transgenic line showing 100 per cent female lethal phenotype has to undergo laboratory cage test and field cage test where the transgenic male insects are released multiple times in weekly interval into the known number of wild or laboratory reared colony insects to see the dwindling number of colony insects after each transgenic male release.

VIII. Nature Release- The Final Step

After clearing all the tests and getting the permission from concerned authorities the transgenic insects will be ready for nature release. The following diagram explains the mode ofoperation of RIDL technology in comparison with SIT to eradicate an insect population.

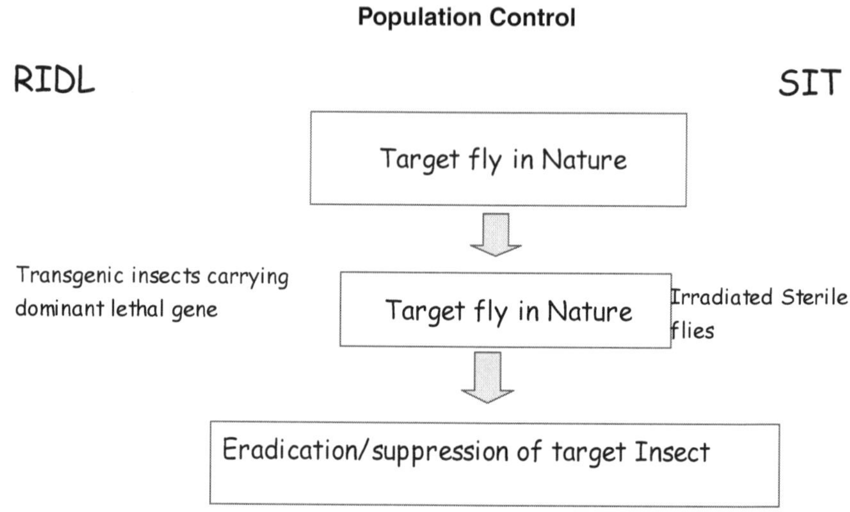

6. Strategies for Genetic Control of Insects

There are two types of genetic control strategies available for population control of insects *viz.* i. Self-limiting strategies and ii. Self-sustaining strategies.

Self-Limiting Strategies

The modification tends to disappear from the target insect population unless replenished by periodic release of additional sterile/GM insects (*e.g.*, SIT, fsRIDL, Bisex-RIDL, IIT, HEGs (autosomal). This strategy is used to suppress the insect population below the economic threshold level. No gene drive and follows Mendelian inheritance of transgenes

Self-Sustaining Strategies

Modification intended to persist indefinitely and perhaps even spread within the initial target insect population or to other populations. (*e.g.*, Transposons, HEGs (Y linked -X chromosome targeting, Underdominance *Wolbachia*). This strategy is proposed for eradication of target insect species. The transgene will be driven into population and follows super-Mendelian inheritance of transgenes.

7. Genetic Control of Screwworm Fly

Cochliomyia hominivorax, New world screwworm (NWS) fly is a subtropical-tropical dipteran insect species of the Americas which causes sever myiasis in animals. Female flies oviposit in wounds of animals as well as humans, and, if untreated, the hatching larvae may cause severe myiasis and death. NWS is successfully eradicated from North and Central America using Sterile Insect Technique. Repeated and programmed release of gamma irradiated screwworm flies into nature led to the eradication of NWS. Screwworm eradication programmewas started by USDA in the year of 1957 under the leadership of Dr. Edward F. Knipling and Dr. Raymond Bushland. In 1982, USA was declared free from NWS flies. USDA extended the NWS eradication programme to Mexico and other central American countries to prevent the re-entry of the flies into USA. In 2006, Panama was declared free from NWS flies. NWS eradication programme costed US$750 and helped to double the cattle population in Texas, USA.The great success of the NWS eradication programme is attributed to the single mating behavior of the female fly, gamma irradiation technology and development artificial diet for laboratory mass rearing.

Steps in SIT of Screwworm

- Mass laboratory rearing of NWS fly
- Radiation mass-sterilization of pupal stage of NWS fly
- Production of reasonably competitive sterile NWS flies
- Assessment of native NWS fly populations before the release of the sterile NWS fly(Capture-recapture-method)
- Releasing and distributing the sterile NWS fly pupae over the treatment area
- Assessment of native NWS fly populations after the release of the sterile NWS fly(Capture-recapture-method)

Selection of sterile insect release area should be large enough (or well-isolated enough to have barrier region) to exclude the possibility of immigration of inseminated females into the release area. Caesium-137 and cobalt-60 radioactive isotopes are commonly used in the ionizing radiation of the NWS flies. A dose of 5500 rad (55 Gy) is sufficient to guarantee 100 per cent sterility of New world screwworm flies and 5 to 6 days-old pupae are used for radiation. Separation of male and female NWS flies is not possible in the conventional sterile insect technique. Male and female pupae are irradiated and released into the nature. Using the **Transgenic Sexing Strains** (TSS) of NWS, it is possible to rear only the male insects and 25Gy of radiation dose is enough to render the male pupae sterile. Release of only the sterile male NWS improves the efficiency of insect population control.

8. Genetic Control of Mosquito

SIT, GM insects technology and IIT are used in the control of mosquito population. GM mosquito approaches is successfully applied to many mosquito species, whereas the success of IIT is based on *Wolbachia*transfection and stable inheritance (*e.g.*, successful in *Ae. aegypti* and *An. stephensi* but difficult in *An. gambiae*). *Wolbachia* population suppression (IIT) and GM mosquito carrying lethal gene approaches have been successfully trialed in several countries. Regulatory hurdles differ substantially between these two methods. Although mosquitoes transfected with *Wolbachia* have not encountered the same regulatory hurdles as GM mosquitoes (*e.g.*, Wolbachia-Mosquitoe are considered "veterinary chemical products" in Australia). At present, GM insects with lethal genes and Wolbachia transfected mosquito with self-limiting strategy (no gene drive) are widely being tested in field for their mosquito population suppression efficiency. Oxitec (Oxford Insect Technology), UK is the company making GM mosquitoes with population suppression strategy. The company successfully conducted several field trials across the globe and reported significant level of wild mosquito population

- Cayman Islands (2009–2010): Male mosquitoes of a RIDL strain of *Ae. aegypti*, OX513A wererereleased and led to strong suppression of the target wild population
- Malaysia (2010): *Ae. aegypti*OX513A males were shown to have similar longevity and maximum dispersal
- French Polynesia (2010): Release of *Ae. polynesiensis* males infected with a *Wolbachia* strain from *Ae. riversi* for IIT trial
- Brazil (2011–2016): sustained release of *Ae. aegypti*OX513A males led to strong suppression of a target wild population.
- Australia (2011–present): Release of Wolbachia wMel-infected male and female *Ae. aegypti* led to the invasion and establishment of wMel*Wolbachia* in two target wild populations
- Vietnam (2013–present): Release of Wolbachia wMelPop-infected male and female *Ae. aegypti* on an island
- USA (2021): Release of Friendly™ *Aedes aegypti* males (GM mosquito eggs in capsule) led to strong suppression of a target wild population.
- Project Wolbachia Singapore (2021-22): male Wolbachia-carrying Aedes aegypti (Wolbachia-Aedes) mosquitoes to reduce the dengue mosquito population

9. Integration into other Pest Management Programs

Hence, SIT and RIDL fit well within the concept of integrated pest management, when combined with other control methods, results in maximum efficiency. The sterile insect release method and RIDL are completely compatible with other types of insect control methods used in IPM programs. These technologies are most efficient and economical when insect populations are already at low levels. *Hematobia irritans*, *Culicoides* spp. midges, *Rhipicephalus microplus* tick and *Phlebotomus* spp. are important arthropod vectors of veterinary importance need to be controlled from diseases endemic areas in India using SIT or RIDL technique to augment the livestock production. Unraveling the factors involved in somatic sex determination pathway of various insects of veterinary importance will give impetus to genetic control of important livestock pests.

REFERENCES

Alan S.Robinson and Gerald Franz (2000) The Application of Transgenic Insect Technology in the Sterile Insect Technique (Chapter 17) in the book Insect Transgenesis: Methods and Applications, Edited by Alfred M. Handler and Anthony James. CRC press. P307-318

Alphey, L. Genetic Control of mosquitoes. *Annu. Rev. Entomol.* 2014. 59: 205–24

Azhahianambi Palavesam, Caroline Esnault and David O'Brochta (2013) Post-integration silencing of *piggyBac* transposable element in *Aedes aegypti.PLoS One*, 8(7): e68454.

Azhahianambi, P and Ghosh,S (2007). Genetic transformation of arthropod vectors for control of vector borne diseases. *Indian Journal of Biotechnology*, 6: 305-314.

Benedict, MQ (Editor) (2014) Transgenic insects: techniques and applications. CABI publications; ISBN 9781780644516, DOI 10.1079/9781780644516.0000

Caroline Esnault, Azhahianambi Palavesam, Kristina Pilitt and David O'Brochta. (2011). Intrinsic characteristics of neighboring DNA modulate transposable element activity in *Drosophila melanogaster*. *Genetics*, 187: 319-331.

Concha C, Azhahianambi Palavesam, Felix D. Guerrero, Sagel An, Li F,Osborne J A,Hernandez Y, Pardo T, Quintero G, Vasquez M, Keller G P, Phillips P L,. Welch J B, McMillan O, Skoda S R and. Scott M J (2016) A transgenic male-only strain of the New World screwworm for an improved control program using the sterile insect technique. *BMC Biology*, 14: 72: DOI 10.1186/s12915-016-0296-8. (PMID: 27576512)

Dyck VA, Hendrichs J, Robinson AS. Sterile insect technique: principles and practice in area-wide integrated pest management. Dordrecht: Springer; 2005

Fu G, Condon KC, Epton MJ, Gong P, Jin L, Condon GC, Morrison NI, Dafa'alla TH, Alphey L. Female-specific insect lethality engineered using alternative splicing. *Nat Biotechnol.* 2007; 25(3): 353–7

O'Brochta DA and Atkinson PW (1997) Recent developments in transgenic insect technology. Parasitol Today,13 (3): 99-104.

Purusothaman, DK., Shackleford, L., Anderson, M.A.E. *et al.*, CRISPR/Cas-9 mediated knock-in by homology dependent repair in the West Nile Virus vector Culex quinquefasciatus Say. *Sci Rep* 11, 14964 (2021

Qiang Xu, Felix D. Guerrero, Azhahianambi Palavesam and Adalberto A. Perez de Leon´ (2015) Use of electroporation as an option to transform the horn fly,

Haematobiairritans: A species recalcitrant to microinjection. *Insect Science* (2015) 00, 1–9, DOI 10.1111/1744-7917.12207

Thomas DD, Donnelly CA, Wood RJ, Alphey LS. Insect population control using a dominant, repressible, lethal genetic system. *Science*. 2000; 287(5462): 2474–6

Van der Vloedt A.M and W. Klassen. The development and application of the sterile insect technique (SIT) for New World screwworm eradication. FAO corporate document repository.http: //www.fao.org/docrep/u4220t/u4220T0j.htm

Chapter 20

Insights into Antiprotozoal Drug Resistance and Ways to a Rational Solution

A.K. Tewari

Division of Parasitology,
ICAR-Indian Veterinary Research Institute,
Izatnagar, Bareilly, Uttar Pradesh

Introduction

The unicellular parasitic protozoa have coevolved with their vertebrate hosts to live in a parasitic association for millions of years. The infections impact the health and productivity of the hosts significantly. The parasitic protozoa have global distribution. The agro-climatic conditions of a geographic area influence the distribution of many pathogenic protozoa spp. and the changes made to the environment and ecology due to the growing human population have influenced the occurrence of several protozoan infections. Although the protozoan parasites are morphologically simple, the metabolic process is complex (Fletcher *et al.*, 2012). Most of the parasitic protozoa are by and large species-specific; the pathogens that cause a life-threatening infection in humans may not be pathogenic at all for the livestock and *vice versa*. For example, *Plasmodium falciparum* though causes a fulminating infection in humans does not cause any clinical disease in the livestock except in the avian species. Similarly, several species of *Eimeria* cause serious enteritis in livestock but do not establish in humans. Nonetheless, several pathogens, *viz. Toxoplasma gondii* can infect both humans and animals alike and cause zoonotic diseases. In nature, the transmission of the infection may occur directly per os or through an invertebrate vector (Inam *et al.*, 2009).

As a protective vaccine is not available for most parasitic infections, chemotherapeutic interventions play a significant role in the mitigation of the impact of diseases. However, the potentially toxic nature of commercially available medicines remains a concern. Moreover, the efficacy of some commercial therapeutic compounds has been compromised due to the development of resistance. The growing concern over widespread drug resistance has underlined the need for developing safer drugs for the therapeutic management of parasitic pathogens. Understanding the biological phenomena that lead to the development of resistance in nature is important to address the issue widespread in human and veterinary medicine and would help identify innovative lead compounds of therapeutic relevance (Capela *et al.*, 2019; Fullybright, 2019).

Drug Resistance

Drug resistance may be defined as the reduction of efficacy of a drug in therapeutic doses. The drug specifically interacts with the target molecule of the pathogen. Any mutation-induced change in the target molecule may contribute to the development of resistance. The therapeutic determinants of an anti-protozoal agent comprise its ability to block the protein synthesis of the pathogen, interfere with the replication and repair of the nucleic acid molecules and block the biosynthesis of major housekeeping enzymes. The resistant pathogen successfully blocks the therapeutic efficacy of the drug leading to increased morbidity and even death of the host. Borst and Ouellette (1995) have reviewed the mechanisms of development of resistance against the anti-protozoal drugs which essentially involve loss of transporter molecules, transmembrane transport proteins, failure of drug activation and alteration of drug targets due to the substitution of amino acids. The decrease in the transporter molecules results in low or no uptake of the drug leading to reduced therapeutic efficacy. This decrease contributes to resistance to arsenicals and diamidines in African trypanosomes. The transmembrane transport proteins, *viz.* P-glycoproteins and other traffic ATPases mediate the export of drugs. Transmembrane transporter-mediated resistance was recorded for emetine, mefloquine and antimonials used for treating *Entamoeba* spp., *Plasmodium* spp., and *Leishmania* spp., respectively. The pfmdr1 gene of *Plasmodium falciparum* might be involved in chloroquine resistance and PgpA P-glycoprotein of *Leishmania* spp. might contribute to resistance to arsenite and antimonials. The failure of drug activation has been ascribed to the resistance against metronidazole in *Trichomonas* and *Giardia* spp. Substitution of amino acids may alter and may contribute to the process of development of resistance. Specific substitutions of amino acid in the dihydrofolate reductase-thymidylate synthase result in the development of resistance in *Plasmodium* spp. through.

Trypanosomosis or Surra

Trypanosoma evansi causes surra and the disease is prevalent in entire south-east Asia and sub-Saharan Africa, while *T. brucei, T. vivax* and *T. congolense* cause animal trypanosomosis in the African continent. Surra occurs as an acute disease in equines and canines, however, chronic infection is more common in the ruminants. The clinical signs of surra are non-specific. Fever, inappetence, anaemia, loss of body mass, poor work capacity, lethargy, abortion, immunosuppression and nervous signs are common. The infection is responsible for huge economic loss due to extensive morbidity and mortality in livestock. The disease is managed therapeutically with a few commercially available drugs of which Diminazene aceturate, isometamidium chloride and quinapyramine compounds are important. Diminazene aceturate and quinapyramine sulphate have a therapeutic effect, while isometamidium chloride and quinapyramine chloride are prophylactic and the protection lasts for about three months (Holmes *et al.*, 2004).

The rapid metabolism and excretion have made diminazene a preferred drug to cure trypanosomosis and babesiosis in livestock (Peregrine and Mamman, 1993). The drug reaches the peak blood level within 1 h of dosing and its elimination follows a biphasic or triphasic behaviour depending on the animal species and formulation. Following intramuscular administration, the elimination of half-life varies from 11–19 h in sheep and goats to 74 to >200 h in cattle (Mamman *et al.*, 1993; Peregrine and Mamman, 1993). Cattle excrete diminazene mainly in the urine (Kellner *et al.*, 1985). Diminazene residues may persist for several weeks in the edible tissues of cattle and other food-producing animals, especially in the liver and kidney, whereas the drug level in milk peak at 6 h and fall below detection limits after 48 h (FAO, 1990). Therefore, pre-slaughter drug withdrawal of 21–35 days is advised for cattle and sheep, while for milk a 3-day discard period is recommended (FAO, 1990; Peregrine and Mamman, 1993).

The trypanocidal mode of action of diminazene is not fully understood. The compound binds the minor groove of the DNA at AT-rich sites (Wilson *et al.*, 2008). In trypanosomes, the kDNA is a known target of the drug, and kDNA binding can cause inhibition of replication and kDNA loss (Shapiro and Englund, 1990). The drug might have an inhibitory effect on mitochondrial type II topoisomerase (Portugal, 1994). The kinetoplast has been resurrected as the potential drug target of diminazene. Diminazene uptake in *T. brucei* occurs via an aminopurine transporter called P2 or *Tb*AT1, which is also implicated in the uptake of the related diamidinepentamidine and the melaminophenyl arsenical melarsoprol, the drugs licensed for HAT (Carter *et al.*, 1995; De Koning, 2008). A P-2 type purine transporter has been shown to involve in the uptake of diminazene aceturate in *T. evansi*. Knocking down or silencing the gene results in resistance (Carter *et al.*, 2005).

Changes in the functional protein conformation may occur due to the dysfunction of a gene and that may lead to drug resistance. The genome-wide RNA interference target sequencing (RIT-seq) identified gene with reduced drug sensitivity in *T. brucei*. The technique identified additional plasma membrane proteins (P-type H^+-ATPases), as well as a putative protein phosphatase, which were related to the pharmacological effect of diamidinepentamidine (Alsford *et al.*, 2012). The key role of the *TbAQP2* gene that codes the HAPT1/*Tb*AQP2 carrier (De Koning, 2001, Baker *et al.*, 2012) in the uptake of pentamidine and the melaminophenyl arsenicals in *T. brucei* is known, however, its role in diminazene uptake is less distinct (Teka *et al.*, 2011; Munday *et al.*, 2014). The loss of P2/*Tb*AT1 is responsible for a high level of resistance to diminazene (Matovu *et al.*, 2003). A mutation in the ATP synthase subunit causes substantial resistance to isometamidium and homidium. The high level of resistance is associated with a loss of mitochondrial membrane potential, preventing further isometamidium accumulation in this organelle (Eze *et al.*, 2016).

Resistance against trypanocidal drugs has been reported in 17 countries of Africa (Delespaux *et al.*, 2008). Isometamidium diffuses through the cytoplasmic membrane of the trypanosome, while the drug enters the mitochondrion by diffusion or by an energy-dependent transmembrane transporter. The resistance against a trypanocidal drug may develop due to lower diffusion through the mitochondrial membrane, modification of a transporter protein located on the mitochondrial membrane, rapid extrusion of the drug from the cytoplasm mediated by a transporter located on the cytoplasmic membrane or by the combination of the processes. There are ubiquitous membrane-bound ABC transporters (ATP-binding cassette) proteins available that transport the substrate across the biomembrane using ATP irrespective of the concentration gradient (Borst and Elfernik, 2002). An amplified fragment length polymorphism study showed insertion of a GAA codon (coding for lysine) in excess in the coding sequence of an ABC transporter conferred resistance against isometamidium in *T. congolense* (Delespaux *et al.*, 2005). However, it is not clear whether the resistance to isometamidium is due to reduced uptake or increased efflux of the drug.

Bovine Tropical Theileriosis

Bovine tropical theileriosis, a tick-borne disease of cattle, is caused by the intracellular protozoan parasite *Theileria annulata*. The disease has a wide prevalence in Southern Europe, Northern Africa and entire Asia. The significant economic loss is associated with the high susceptibility of exotic and crossbred cattle and can cause 40–50 per cent mortality if the animals are left untreated (Gharbi *et al.*, 2011; Brown, 1990).

Buparvaquone (trans-2-[4-(4-butyl cyclohexyl methyl)]-3-hydroxy-1, 4-naphthoquinone) has been the drug of choice for the treatment of tropical bovine theileriosis, caused by *T. annulata* since its introduction in the late 1980s. The drug has a high therapeutic index and low toxicity to cattle. However, there are several reports on the development of resistance against the drug. The infection caused either mortality or a persistently high level of parasitemia in the survivors despite an early treatment with a conventional dose of the drug (2.5 mg/kg) (Mhadhbi *et al.*, 2010).

Although the mechanism of action of buparvaquone has not been fully elucidated, the naphthoquinones are known to cause competitive inhibition of the ubiquinone binding (coenzyme Q) to cytochrome b of the mitochondrial cytochrome bc1 complex leading to the inhibition of electron transport and the collapse of mitochondrial membrane potential (Fry and Pudney, 1992). Mhadhavi*et al.* (2015) showed that resistance of *T. annulata* to buparvaquone was associated with mutations in the functional drug binding regions Q_0cytb gene region. Hacilarlioglu *et al.* (2012) analysed the *Theileria annulata* isolates, collected from the clinical cases of drug-resistant tropical theileriosis. The authors reported two nonsynonymous mutations at positions 135 and 253 that resulted in the substitution of valine to alanine and from proline to serine, respectively. The change in the hydrophobicity due to the substitution explains the decreased affinity of buparvaquone to cytochrome b. The use of a low dose of the drug for therapy and the selection pressure generated due to the massive use of buparvaquone in the field during the last more than thirty years might have contributed to the emergence of resistance.

Babesiosis

Several species of *Babesia*, the intraerythrocytic apicomplexan parasite, are known to cause fatal infection in livestock. The disease is characterised by high fever, and anaemia leading to significant morbidity. Mortality in absence of specific chemotherapeutic intervention may occur. *Babesia bigemina* causes red water fever in bovines, while *B. canis* and *B. gibsoni* are associated with clinical babesiosis in canines. The parasites are widely distributed in India and other tropical countries. There are sizeable reports that exist on the development of drug resistance in *Babesia* species (Hwang *et al.*, 2010; Yamasaki *et al.*, 2017). Development of resistance to diminazene aceturate has been reported in *Babesia bovis* (Tuvshintulga *et al.*, 2019).

In vivo Methods for Detection of Drug Resistance

Assessment of the level of resistance is crucial for successful treatment and control of the infection. However, it is difficult to develop reliable tests for widespread use in the endemic zones. To identify drug resistance in the field, the 'block treatment' approach was proposed (Delespaux *et al.*, 2008). The method relies on the comparison of time to detect the parasite in the treated and the untreated controls (Eisler *et al.*, 2000). Smaller the difference correlated to the likely chance of the development of resistance. The method is time and cost-intensive and requires sizeable numbers of target animals, like cattle, to get an indication of resistance. The confirmation of the drug efficacy relies primarily on infection and treatment experiments involving the natural hosts or laboratory animals. The clearance of parasites is assessed by a suitable test like microscopy (Eisler *et al.,* 2001). The method is cumbersome, expensive and requires a long follow-up period. In the field condition, the chance of reinfection after successful treatment remains and that may lead to an erroneous conclusion. The extrapolation of rodent data to ruminants is not necessarily an accurate reflection of treatment success in large animals (Eisler *et al.,* 2001). Nevertheless, the single-dose mouse test is currently considered the standard test to study single or multiple resistance in *T. congolense* and *T. brucei* isolates at an accelerated rate. The drug sensitivity studies in rodents can be improved by substituting microscopy with PCR based detection methods (Tran *et al.,* 2014).

In vitro Methods for Detection of Drug Resistance

Large scale *in vitro* cultivation techniques facilitated the search for new lead compounds and assessment of their sensitivity, especially in the bloodstream form *salivarian trypanosomes* (Diaz et *al.,* 2014). The *in vitro* culture techniques made a quick determination of the drug sensitivity of the new lead molecules possible in a cost-effective way than the *in vivo* tests (Kaminsky and Brun, 1993). The assays include Alamar blue test (Räz *et al.,*1997), the drug incubation infectivity test (DIIT) (Kaminsky *et al.,*1990) and the [^{3}H] hypoxanthine incorporation test (Brun and Kunz, 1989). The latter two tests evaluate the viability of the parasite, following 24 h exposure to drug dilutions in a culture medium, by their ability to infect mice or incorporate tritiated hypoxanthine. The drug incubation *Glossina* infectivity test (DIGIT) (Clausen *et al.,*1999) relies on the ability of the trypanosomes to infect tsetse flies following an *in vitro* exposure to specific doses of trypanocidal drugs.

Molecular Methods for Detection of Drug Resistance

Single-Strand Conformation Polymorphism (SSCP)

The SSCP is an important diagnostic tool in molecular biology. The technique may be defined as a conformational difference of single-stranded nucleotide sequences of identical length which is induced by differences in the sequences under certain experimental conditions. Electrophoretic separation of fragments, according to their different conformations allows sequences to be distinguished. SSCP is used in genotyping to detect homozygous individuals of different allelic states, as well as heterozygous individuals that should each demonstrate distinct patterns in an electrophoresis experiment (Oto *et al.,* 1993).

Polymerase Chain Reaction-Restriction Fragment Length Polymorphism (PCR RFLP)

If the locus of a gene is occupied by more than one allele, and the rate of distribution is more than 1 per cent in the population, the gene is referred to as polymorphic. Gene polymorphisms can occur in any region of the genome. The majority of polymorphisms are silent and do not alter the function or expression of a gene, a polymorphic variant of a gene can have an abnormal expression which can produce an abnormal form of a protein with a serious consequence. Restriction fragment length polymorphism (RFLP) exploits the polymorphisms of the genetic sequence to distinguish individuals, populations or species. To detect polymorphisms, a DNA sample is digested by one or more restriction enzymes and the resulting restriction fragments are separated by agar gel electrophoresis based on their size.

Single Nucleotide Polymorphism (SNP)

The single nucleotide polymorphism is a single base-pair mutation at a specific locus and measures the variation between the members of a species. Since the SNPs are evolutionarily conserved, they are used as a marker for quantitative trait loci analysis and in association studies.

Allele-Specific PCR (AS PCR)

Kary Mullis described the technique of *in vitro* amplification of target DNA fragments through the polymerase chain reaction (PCR) in 1983. Later C. R. Newton and coworkers described the allele-specific PCR for the detection of mutations like deletion, duplications, insertion or SNP. Alleles are the alternative forms of a gene. A mutation gives rise to two different forms of a gene- a normal and another mutant. The AS PCR can detect a specific allele and that is made possible by the introduction of minor changes in the primers. The 3′end of the primer is modified in a way that one primer recognises the normal allele while the other recognises the mutant. Several molecular methods have extensively been used for the detection of drug sensitivity. The PCR-based techniques were used to assess the status of alleles responsible for drug resistance (Kazibwe *et al.*,2009; Graf *et al.*,2013). Resistance to melaminophenyl arsenicals and diamidines has been ascribed to mutations in the *TbAT1* and *TbAQP2* genes (Graf *et al.*, 2015). The development of diminazene resistance was ascribed to the mutation of the *TbAT1* gene of*T. b. evansi* and *T. b. equiperdum* (Barrett *et al.*,1995; Stewart *et al.*, 2010). Resistance to the eflornithine, used for the treatment of human African trypanosomiasis was related to the loss of the amino acid transporter *Tb*AAT6 (Vincent *et al.*, 2010; Schumann *et al.*, 2011; Alsford *et al.*, 2012).

Besides the genetic tests, fluorescence-based tests have also been used to assess the presence or absence of the transporter proteins, *viz.* P2/*Tb*AT1 (Stewart *et al.*, 2005). However, there are no reliable markers identified to assess the drug resistance in *T. congolense* and *T. vivax*. To detect the polymorphism in an ABC-type multidrug transporter putative gene related to isometamidium resistance in *T. congolense*, the *Mbo*II–PCR–RFLP was exploited (Delespaux *et al.*, 2005). The sensitive strain showed a polymorphism at the 381 bp fragment, whereas the resistant strain showed it at the 384 bp fragment of a putative gene that showed some homology with the ABC transporter (Delespaux*et al.*, 2005).

A simple *Bcl*I-PCR-RFLP test was developed based on the single-strand conformation polymorphism (SSCP) analysis of the *T. congolense* P2-type purine transporter *Tco*AT1 for the rapid identification of Diminazene (DA)-resistant stocks (V. Delespaux, *et al.*,2006). The test was based on a single nucleotide replacement (G to A) in the DA-resistant strains. This single point mutation confers the replacement of Valto Ile at position 306 in the purine transporter. A set of six conserved point mutations was described in the *Tb*AT1 gene of melarsoprol-resistant *T. brucei* strains (Mäsere *t al.*,1999). Further, detection of DA resistance in *T. brucei* isolates was attempted with *Sfa*NI polymorphism studies together with AS-PCR (Nerima, *et al.*2008). The study showed that the finding of AS-PCR correlated 100 per cent with *Sfa*NI-PCR-RFLP. The advantage of the test relied on its less expensiveness and time efficiency than *Sfa*NI-PCR-RFLP.

Other Methods for Detection of Drug Resistance

An isometamidium (ISM)-ELISA was described to detect the isometamidium resistance in trypanosomes. The test is based on the variation of mitochondrial electrical potential (MEP) which determines the rate of ISM accumulation in the trypanosome kinetoplast (Wilkes *et al.*, 1997). Preliminary studies on *T. congolense* showed that the MEP could be a candidate marker for ISM resistance studies. An ELISA was standardised to detect serum ISM and combined with the test to screen the resistant trypanosomes (Eisler *et al.*, 1996). The trypanosomes that survived in the animals with ISM serum concentrations above 0.4ng per ml were considered resistant (Eisler *et al.*, 1997).

How to Overcome the Complex Issue of Drug Resistance?

Identification of several molecular markers for anti-protozoal drug resistance has made it possible to identify the drug-resistance genes and their stability after withdrawal of the drug selection pressure. This has contributed immensely to our understanding of the epidemiology of drug resistance. Although the molecular markers help in the faster detection of resistance, the process is complex. The active transportation of the drug through biological membranes is specific and may involve several pathways for the importers or extruders. To delineate the process, several diagnostic tests are required. Moreover, there may be more than one process involved in conferring resistance, *viz.* isometamidium resistance might be caused by a synergistic combination of reduced uptake and increased efflux of the drug. A careful study of the level of expression of the genes coding for the importers or extruders, as well as the determination of the number of copies of a gene coding each transporter is essential for the identification of the resistant phenotypes. Recent techniques like CRISPR CAS9 and qPCR might help in understanding the process. However, the persistent requirement of live parasites for an effective outcome of these techniques constitutes the major constraint, besides the cost and human factors involved.

To put an effective check on the development of drug resistance, a holistic approach involving all the stakeholders of human and veterinary medicine is essential. To achieve the goal, a stewardship program to restrict and reduce the use of licenced drugs and its strict implementation is critical. Judicious application of the drugs in the right doses under appropriate supervision needs to be made mandatory with a check on the over the counter sale of the licenced drugs. An international effort is needed to check the growing menace.

REFERENCES

Alsford, S., Eckert, S., Baker, N., Glover, L., Sanchez-Flores, A., Leung, K. F., Turner, D. J., Field, M.C., Berriman, M. and Horn, D. High-throughput decoding of antitrypanosomal drug efficacy and resistance. Nature 2012. 482, 232–236.

Baker, N., Glover, L., Munday, J.C., Aguinaga, A.D., Barrett, M.P., deKoning, H.P. and Horn, Aquaglyceroporin 2 controls susceptibility to melarsoprol and pentamidine in African trypanosomes. Proceedings of the National Academy of Sciences of the United States of America 2012. 109, 10996–11001.

Barrett, M.P., Zhang, Z.Q., Denise, H., Giroud, C. and Baltz, T. A.Diamidineresistant *Trypanosoma equiperdum* clone contains a P2 purine transporter with reduced substrate affinity. Molecular and Biochemical Parasitology 1995. 73, 223–229.

Borst P, Ouellette M. New mechanisms of drug resistance in parasitic protozoa. Annu Rev Microbiol. 1995; 49: 427-60. DOI: 10.1146/annurev.mi.49.100195.002235. PMID: 8561467.

Borst, P. and Elfernik, R.O. Mammalian ABC transporters in health and disease. 2002; Ann. Rev. Biochem, 71: 537-592.

Brown, C. G. Control of tropical theileriosis (*Theileria annulata* infection) of cattle. *Parassitologia* 1990. 32: 23–31.

Brun, R. and Kunz, C. *In vitro* drug sensitivity test for *Trypanosoma brucei* subgroup bloodstream trypomastigotes. ActaTropica1989. 46, 361–368.

Capela R, Moreira R, Lopes F. An Overview of Drug Resistance in Protozoal Diseases. Int J Mol Sci. 2019 20(22): 5748. DOI: 10.3390/ijms20225748. PMID: 31731801; PMCID: PMC6888673.

Carter, N S *et al.*, Uptake of diamidine drugs by the P2 nucleoside transporter in melarsen sensitive and resistant *Trypanosomabruceibrucei.* 2005 J Biol Chem. 270: 28153-28157.

Carter, N. S., Berger, B. J. and Fairlamb, A. H. Uptake of diamidine drugs by the P2 nucleoside transporter in melarsen-sensitive and -resistant *Trypanosoma bruceibrucei*. J. Biol. Chem. 1995. 270, 28153-28157.

Clausen, P.H., Leendertz, F.H., Blankenburg, A., Tietjen, U., Mehlitz, D., Sidibe, I. and Bauer, B. A drug incubation glossina infectivity test (DIGIT) to assess the susceptibility of *Trypanosoma congolense* bloodstream forms to trypanocidal drugs (Xenodiagnosis). Acta Trop.1999. 72, 111–117.

De Koning, H. P. Ever-increasing complexities of diamidine and arsenical cross-resistance in African trypanosomes. Trends Parasitol. 2008. 24, 345–349.

De Koning, H. P. Uptake of pentamidine in *Trypanosoma brucebrucei* is mediated by three distinct transporters: implications for cross-resistance with arsenicals. Mol. Pharmacol. 2001. 59, 586–592.

Delespaux*et al.,* Identification of a genetic marker for isometamidium chloride resistance in *Trypanosoma congolense.* Int. J. Parasitol. 2005. 35: 235-243.

Delespaux V, Geysen D, Van den Bossche P, Geerts S. Molecular tools for the rapid detection of drug resistance in animal trypanosomes. Trends Parasitol. 2008 24(5): 236-42. doi: 10.1016/j.pt.2008.02.006.

Delespaux, V., Geysen, D., VandenBossche, P. and Geerts, S. Molecular tools for the rapid detection of drug resistance in animal trypanosomes. Trends Parasitol. 2005. 24, 236–242.

Diaz, R., Luengo-Arratta, S. A., Seixas, J. D., Amata, E., Devine, W., Cordon-Obras, C., Rojas-Barros, D. I., Jimenez, E., Ortega, F., Crouch, S., Colmenarejo, G., Fiandor, J. M., Martin, J.J., Berlanga, M., Gonzalez, S., Manzano, P., Navarro, M. and Pollastri, M. P. (Identification and characterization of hundreds of potent and selective inhibitors of *Trypanosoma brucei* growth from a kinase-targeted library screening campaign. PLoS Neglected Tropical Diseases 2014. 8, e3253.

Eisler, M.C. *et al.,* Concentrations of isometamidium in the sera of cattle challenged with drug-resistant *Trypanosoma congolense.* Acta Trop. 1997. 63. 89-100.

Eisler, M.C. *et al., A* simple competitive enzyme immunoassay for the detection of the trypanocidal drug isometamidium. Ther. Drug Monit. 1996. 18. 73-79.

Eisler, M.C., Brandt, J., Bauer, B., Clausen, P.H., Delespaux, V., Holmes, P.H., Ilemobade, A., Machila, N., Mbwambo, H., McDermott, J., Mehlitz, D., Murilla, G., Ndung'u, J.M., Peregrine, A. S., Sidibe, I., Sinyangwe, L. and Geerts, S. Standardised tests in mice and cattle for the detection of drug resistance in tsetse-transmitted trypanosomes of African domestic cattle. Vet. Parasitol. 2001. 97, 171–182.

Eisler, M.C., McDermott, J.J., Mdachi, R., Murilla, G.A., Sinyangwe, L., Mubanga, J., Machila, N., Mbwambo, H., Coleman, P.G., Clausen, P.H., Bauer, B., Sidibé, I., Geerts, S., Holmes, P. H. and Peregrine, A. S. Rapid method for the assessment of trypanocidal drug resistance in the field. In *Proceedings of the 9th Symposium of the International Society for Veterinary Epidemiology and Economics*, Nairobi, Kenya, paper 2000. 353 1–3.

Eze, A.A., Gould, M.K., Munday, J.C., Tagoe, D., Stelmanis, V., Schnaufer, A.C. and de Koning, H. P. Loss of mitochondrial membrane potential is a late adaptation of *Trypanosoma bruceibrucei* to isometamidium preceded by mutations in the γ subunit of the F_1F_0-ATPase. PLoS Neglected Tropical Diseases 2016. 10, e0004791.

FAO. Residues of Some Veterinary Drugs in Animals and Foods. FAO Food and Nutrition 1990. paper No. 41/2. Food and Agriculture Organization of the United Nations (FAO), Rome, Italy.

Fletcher S.M., Stark D., Harkness J., Ellisa J. Enteric Protozoa in the Developed World: A Public Health Perspective. *Clin. Microbiol. Rev.* 2012; 25: 420–449. DOI: 10.1128/CMR.05038-11.

Fry M, Pudney M. Site of action of the antimalarial dihydroxynaphthoquinone, 2-[trans-4-(4′-chlorophenyl)cyclohexyl]-3-hydroxy-1,4-naphthoquinone (566C80). *Biochem Pharmacol.* 1992. 43: 1545–1553.

Fullybright R. Characterization of Biological Resistance and Successful Drug Resistance Control in Medicine. Pathogens. 2019; 8: 73. DOI: 10.3390/pathogens8020073. PMID: 31159292; PMCID: PMC6631572.

Gharbi M, Touay A, Khayeche M, Laarif J, Jedidi M, Sassi L, *et al.*, Ranking control options for tropical theileriosis in at-risk dairy cattle in Tunisia, using benefit-cost analysis. *Rev Sci Tech* 2011. 30: 763–778.

Graf, F.E., Baker, N., Munday, J.C., de Koning, H.P., Horn, D. and Maser, P. Chimerization at the AQP2-AQP3 locus is the genetic basis of melarsoprol-pentamidine cross-resistance in clinical *Trypanosoma bruceigambiense* isolates. Int. J. Parasitol.-Drug. 2015.5, 65–68.

Graf, F.E., Ludin, P., Wenzler, T., Kaiser, M., Brun, R., Pyana, P.P., Buscher, P., de Koning, H. P., Horn, D. and Maser, P. Aquaporin 2 mutations in *Trypanosoma bruceigambiense* field isolates correlate with decreased susceptibility to pentamidine and melarsoprol. PLoS Neglected Tropical Diseases 2013. 7, e2475.

Hacilarlioglu S, Bilgic HB, Bakirci S, Weir W, Tait A, Unlu AH, Karagenç T (2012) Are mutations in the cytochrome b gene of *Theileria annulata* responsible for resistance to the theilericidal drug, Buparvaquone? Joint conference on emerging and re-emerging epidemics affecting global health. Orvieto, Italy, September 19–22, 2012.

Holmes P.H. *et al.*, Current chemotherapy of animal trypanosomiasis. (Maudlin, I. Holmes, P H and Miles, M A eds) pp 431-444, CABI Publishing.

Hwang S.J., Yamasaki M., Nakamura K., Sasaki N., Murakami M., WickramasekaraRajapakshage B.K., Ohta H., Maede Y., Takiguchi M. Development and characterization of a strain of *Babesia gibsoni* resistant to diminazene aceturate *in vitro*. *J. Vet. Med. Sci.* 2010; 72: 765–771

Imam T.S. The Complexities in the Classification of Protozoa: A Challenge to Parasitologists. *Bayero J. Pure Appl. Sci.* 2009; 2: 159–164. DOI: 10.4314/bajopas.v2i2.63805.

Kaminsky, R. and Brun, R. *In vitro* assays to determine drug sensitivities of African trypanosomes: a review. Acta Trop. 1993. 54, 279–289.

Kaminsky, R., Gumm, I. D., Zweygarth, E. and Chuma, F. A drug incubation infectivity test (DIIT) for assessing resistance in trypanosomes. Vet. Parasitol.1990. 34, 335–343.

Kazibwe, A.J., Nerima, B., de Koning, H. P., Maser, P., Barrett, M. P. and Matovu, E. Genotypic status of the TbAT1/P2 adenosine transporter of *Trypanosoma bruceigambiense* isolates from Northwestern Uganda following melarsoprol withdrawal. PLoS Neglected Tropical Diseases 2009. 3, e523.

Kellner, H. M., Eckert, H. G. and Volz, M. H. Studies in cattle on the disposition of the anti-trypanosomal drug diminazenediaceturate (Berenil). Trop. Med. Parasitol. 1985. 36, 199–204.

Mamman, M., Aliu, Y. O. and Peregrine, A. S. Comparative pharmacokinetics of diminazene in noninfectedBoran (*Bosindicus*) cattle and Boran cattle infected with *Trypanosoma congolense*. Antimicrob. Agents Chemother. 1993. 37, 1050–1055.

Mäser, P.*et al.*, A nucleoside transporter from *Trypanosoma brucei* involved in drug resistance. Science 1999.285, 242-244

Matovu, E., Stewart, M.L., Geiser, F., Brun, R., Maser, P., Wallace, L.J., Burchmore, R.J., Enyaru, J. C., Barrett, M. P., Kaminsky, R., Seebeck, T. and de Koning, H. P. Mechanisms of arsenical and diamidine uptake and resistance in *Trypanosoma brucei*. Eukaryot. Cell2003. 2, 1003–1008.

Matsuu A., Miyamoto K., Ikadai H., Okano S., Higuchi S. Short report: cloning of the *Babesia gibsoni* cytochrome B gene and isolation of three single nucleotide polymorphisms from parasites present after atovaquone treatment. Am. J. Trop. Med. Hyg. 2006; 74: 593–597

Mhadhbi M, Naouach A, Boumiza A, Chaabani MF, BenAbderazzak S, Darghouth MA In vivo evidence for the resistance of *Theileria annulata* to buparvaquone. Vet Parasitol.2010. 169: 241–247. 10.1016/j.vetpar.2010.01.013

Mhadhbi, M., Chaouch, M., Ajroud, K., Darghouth, M. A., and BenAbderrazak, S. Sequence Polymorphism of Cytochrome b Gene in Theileria annulata Tunisian Isolates and Its Association with Buparvaquone Treatment Failure. PloS one, 2015.10, e0129678. https: //doi.org/10.1371/journal.pone.0129678

Munday, J. C., Eze, A. A., Baker, N., Glover, L., Clucas, C., Aguinaga, A. D., Natto, M. J., Teka, I. A., McDonald, J., Lee, R. S., Graf, F. E., Ludin, P., Burchmore, R. J., Turner, C.M., Tait, A., MacLeod, A., Maser, P., Barrett, M.P., Horn, D. and deKoning, H. P. *Trypanosoma brucei* aquaglyceroporin 2 is a high-affinity transporter for pentamidine and melaminophenyl arsenic drugs and the main genetic determinant of resistance to these drugs. J. Antimicrob. Chemother.2014. 69, 651–663.

Nerima, B. *et al.*, Detection of mutant P2 Adenosine transporter (TbAT1) gene in *T. b. gambiense* isolates from Northwest Uganda using Allele-specific PCR. Trop. Med. Int. Health. 2008. 12, 1361-1368

Oto, M, Miyake, S and Yasuhito Yuasa "Optimization of Nonradioisotopic Single-Strand Conformation Polymorphism Analysis with a Conventional Minislab Gel Electrophoresis Apparatus". Anal. Biochem. 1993. 213: 19–22. doi: 10.1006/abio.1993.1379

Peregrine, A. S. and Mamman, M. Pharmacology of diminazene: a review. Acta Trop. 1993 54, 185–203.

Portugal, J. Berenil acts as a poison of eukaryotic topoisomerase II. FEBS Letters1994. 344, 136–138.

Räz, B., Iten, M., Grether-Buhler, Y., Kaminsky, R. and Brun, R. The Alamar Blue® assay to determine drug sensitivity of African trypanosomes (*T. b. rhodesiense* and *T.b. gambiense*) *in vitro*. Acta Trop.1997. 68, 139–147.

Schumann, B. G., Jutzi, P. and Roditi, I. Genome-wide RNAi screens in bloodstream-form trypanosomes identify drug transporters. MolBiochem. Parasitol. 2011. 175, 91–94.

Shapiro, T. A. and Englund, P. T. Selective cleavage of kinetoplast DNA minicircles promoted by antitrypanosomal drugs. PNAS (USA). 1990. 87, 950–954.

Stewart, M. L., Krishna, S., Burchmore, R. J., Brun, R., de Koning, H. P., Boykin, D. W., Tidwell, R. R., Hall, J. E. and Barrett, M. P. Detection of arsenical drug resistance in *Trypanosoma brucei* with a simple fluorescence test. Lancet 2005. 366, 486–487.

Stewart, M.L., Burchmore, R.J., Clucas, C., HertzFowler, C., Brooks, K., Tait, A., MacLeod, A., Turner, C. M., de Koning, H. P., Wong, P. E. and Barrett, M. P. Multiple genetic mechanisms lead to loss of functional TbAT1 expression in drug-resistant trypanosomes. Eukaryot. Cell 2010. 9, 336–343.

Teka, I. A., Kazibwe, A. J., El-Sabbagh, N., Al-Salabi, M. I., Ward, C. P., Eze, A. A., Munday, J. C., Maser, P., Matovu, E., Barrett, M. P. and de Koning, H. P. The diamidinediminazene aceturate is a substrate for the high-affinity pentamidine transporter: implications for the development of high resistance levels in trypanosomes. Mol. Pharmacol. 2011. 80, 110–116.

Tran, T., Napier, G., Rowan, T., Cordel, C., Labuschagne, M., Delespaux, V., VanReet, N., Erasmus, H., Joubert, A. and Buscher, P. Development and evaluation of an ITS1 "Touchdown" PCR for assessment of drug efficacy against animal African trypanosomosis. Vet. Parasitol. 2014. 202, 164–170.

Tuvshintulga, B., Sivakumar, T., Yokoyama, N. and Igarashi, I.Development of unstable resistance to diminazene aceturate in *Babesia bovis*.Int J Parasitol-Drugs. 2019. 87–92. DOI: 10.1016/j.ijpddr.2019.02.001

V. Delespaux, *et al.*, SCP analysis of the P2 purine transporter TcoAT1 gene of *Trypanosoma congolense* leads to a simple PCR-RFLP test allowing the rapid identification of diminazene resistant stocks Acta Trop. 2006. 100. 96-102

Vincent, I. M., Creek, D., Watson, D. G., Kamleh, M. A., Woods, D. J., Wong, P. E., Burchmore, R. J. and Barrett, M. P. A molecular mechanism for eflornithine resistance in African trypanosomes. PLoS Pathogens. 2010. 6, e1001204.

Wilkes, J.M. *et al.*, Modulation of mitochondrial electrical potential: a candidate mechanism for drug resistance in African trypanosomes. Biochem. J., 1997. 326. 755-761

Wilson, W.D., Tanious, F.A., Mathis, A., Tevis, D., Hall, J.E. and Boykin, D.W. (2008). Antiparasitic compounds that target DNA. Biochimie 90, 999–1014.

Yamasaki M., Watanabe N., Idaka N., Yamamori T., Otsuguro K., Uchida N., Iguchi A., Ohta H., Takiguchi M. Intracellular diminazene aceturate content and adenosine incorporation in diminazene aceturate-resistant *Babesia gibsoni* isolate *in vitro*. *Exp. Parasitol.* 2017; 183: 92–98.

Chapter 21

Anticoccidial Drug Resistance in Ruminants and its Mitigation Strategies

R. Verma, G. Das, S. Kumar, S. Nath, N. Muwel, R.K. Khare, S. Sachan and V. Punia

College of Veterinary Science and Animal Husbandry, NDVSU, Jabalpur – 482 001, Madhya Pradesh

Introduction

Animal husbandry is one of the most important economic activities in the rural areas of the country and contributing significantly to national economy. It generates income for agriculturally dependent households as well as many landless households. Livestock also serves as a source of protein in the form of milk, eggs, and meat. According to 20th livestock census, total livestock population in the India is 536.76 million and has increase by 4.8 per cent as compared to the previous census. Livestock rearing has grown in popularity in recent decades due to its favourable economic prospects, particularly in an intensive and semi-intensive system for mass production. These farming systems significantly increase the risk of coccidiosis in animals, resulting in significant economic losses for farmers because the disease is mostly subclinical and most animals do not exhibit symptoms. Coccidiosis is an intestinal disease caused by protozoan parasites of the genus *Eimeria*, subfamily Eimeriinae of the phylum Apicomplexa (Barta *et al.*, 2001). The disease is more predominant in confined animals kept in intensive husbandry practises (Chhabra and Pandey, 1991). The disease is spread by ingesting sporulated oocysts in contaminated feed or water, or by licking contaminated surfaces. The severity of the disease is determined by the amount of sporulated oocysts consumed; as more oocysts are consumed, the disease becomes worse. Several factors influence disease distribution and prevalence, including sudden changes in weather or extreme weather conditions, higher stock densities, poor hygiene, feed change, feed quality, and any other factor that compromises disease resistance and general health status of the animal. This parasite causes significant economic losses due to intestine lining damage, resulting in decreased appetite, decreased body weight, impaired feed conversion, unthriftiness, diarrhoea, dysentery, anaemia, and increased susceptibility to other diseases. A number of *Eimeria* species have been identified in different animals, but only a few are pathogenic, as shown in Table 21.1. To date identification of *Eimeria* species are based mainly on oocysts morphological characteristics under microscopic examination, parasite biology, clinical signs in the affected animals and typical macroscopic lesions assessed by lesion scores. However, due to the presence of intraspecies variation, the morphological method is not fully reliable since natural infections by *Eimeria* are generally mixed with more than one species and several species have confusing features. Furthermore, morphological observations combined with faecal examination are very labour-intensive and require a skilful classification technique. Molecular approaches have been developed to differentiate between the species of *Eimeria* in goats targeting different regions of the *Eimeria* genome such as internal transcribed spacer-1 (ITS-1) (Verma *et al.*, 2017), small subunit rRNA (Khodakaram *et al.*, 2013), and COI genes (Al-Habsi *et al.*, 2017; Bawm *et al.*, 2020). The control of ruminant coccidiosis is traditionally based on the combination of good management together with prophylacticor metaphylactic treatment with anticoccidials (Daugschies and Najdrowski, 2015). Anticoccidial resistance (ACR) is a widely recognised problem in poultry production (McDougald *et al.*, 1987; Peek and Landman, 2005; Lan *et al.*, 2017). However, despite the widespread use of anticoccidials in mammals, anticoccidial resistance has been not yet been documented in India and only few studies have been reported in abroad (porcine (Sheresta *et al.*, 2017), ovine (Odden *et al.*, 2018), caprine *Eimeria* species (Paul and Sharma, 2014; Hsieh *et al.*, 2020). On the other hand, parasites can potentially generate resistance for chemical anti-coccidial drugs due to bad practices in use. Furthermore, drugs and antibiotic residues in meat is potentially annoyance to consumer. Therefore, the present chapter

Table 21.1: Most Pathogenic *Eimeria* Species infecting in different Animals

S. No.	Animal	Most pathogenic *Eimeria* species
1.	Cattle	*E. zuernii, E. bovis & E. alabamensis*
2	Buffalo	*E. bareillyi, E. bovis & E. zuernii*
3	Sheep	*E. ahsata, E. ovinoidalis & E. crandalis*
4	Goat	*E. arloingi, E. ninakohlyakimovae & E. christenseni*

looks at the current status of anticoccidial drug resistance in ruminants along with mitigation strategies.

Diagnosis of *Eimeria* Species

Based on History and Clinical Symptoms

Overcrowding, poor hygiene, bad weather, animal age (lambs and kids are especially vulnerable between the ages of 3 and 6 months, and calves between the ages of 6 and 12 months), poor growth rate, and sudden death during the weaning period should all be considered indicators of coccidiosis. The most common symptom is diarrhoea, which can be hemorrhagic in sheep but is less common than in cattle (Foreyt, 1990). In contrast, diarrhoea in kids is never hemorrhagic. The faeces are watery with clumps of mucus and range in colour from brown to yellow or dark tarry (Koudela and Bokova, 1998). Dehydration, weight loss/reduced weight gain, and pale mucus membrane are also clinical symptoms associated with diarrhoea.

Post-mortem and Histopathology Lesions

Coccidiosis gross lesions vary depending on the host species, parasite species, and intestinal location. Lesions in sheep and goats vary from proliferative to necrotic-hemorrhagic in cattle, avian species, dogs, and cats. The most common lesions of clinical coccidiosis in young sheep and goats are scattered whitish non-pedunculated plaques to nodules on mucosa of small intestines. The histopathology of lesions in affected animal showed papillary hyperplasia of the epithelium with the presence of intracellular developmental stages of *Eimeria* along with inflammatory cells in the entire intestine.

Faecal Examination

The presence or absence of *Eimeria* oocysts in a faecal sample is determined using the McMaster technique, and the number of oocysts per gram (OPG) of faeces is calculated. Other copromicroscopical techniques also used to determine the OPG by the FLOTAC, mini-FLOTAC and FECPAK (Coles, 2003; Cringoli *et al.*, 2010; Bosco *et al.*, 2014). However, recent reports suggested that the Mini-FLOTAC technique is more sensitive than McMaster egg counting, particularly in small ruminants (Silva *et al.*, 2013; Vieira *et al.*, 2021). Normal animals commonly shed a small number of oocysts. Counts of 5000 oocysts per gram or higher, combined with a typical clinical picture, are strongly suggestive of coccidiosis in cattle and buffalo. However, more than 50,000 oocysts per gram in small ruminants are more highly pathogenic (Verma *et al.*, 2016, 2018). Speciation of the oocysts is important because a large number of non-pathogenic species can be found in animals suffering from other diarrheal diseases. Clinical signs can also appear in the early stages of the disease when faecal shedding is low, or in animals with intestinal scarring who are in the chronic stages of the disease. For specification, oocysts are harvested from a positive faecal sample using a simple floatation method with NaCl as the floating solution. Salt from isolated oocysts will be separated by washing with distilled water/buffer for 2-3 times. Oocysts suspension will be centrifuged and adjusted to a desired précised concentrate. The worked oocysts are for sporulation by 2-2.5 per cent solution of potassium dichromate at room temperature for 7-10 days. The sporulated oocysts to examined under 400× magnifications (one 10× ocular lens and one 40× objective lens) to identify the species based on their sizes and morphological characteristics (shape, colour, form index, presence or absence of micropyle and its cap, presence or absence of residual, polar and stieda bodies) of the oocysts and sporocysts (Pellérdy, 1974; Levine, 1985; Soulsby, 1986; Wang *et al.*, 1990). Approximately 50-100 sporulated/unsporulated oocysts from each species, tentatively identified have take up for micrometry to assist identification of various *Eimeria* species (Levine, 1978; Norton, 1986).

Molecular Techniques

Most of the molecular studies have been conducted on poultry coccidiosis by using various polymerase chain reaction (PCR) assays for species differentiation of *Eimeria* targeting different regions of the *Eimeria* genome like first internal transcribed spacer-1(ITS-1) (Schnitzler *et al.*, 1998), second internal transcribed spacers of ribosomal DNA (ITS-2) (Gasser *et al.*, 2001) and small subunit rRNA (Tsuji *et al.*, 1999). ITS sequences have been used as genetic markers for the identification of species in various organisms including *Eimeria* (Mugridge *et al.*, 2000). The internal transcribed spacer1 (ITS1) region derived from the ribosomal RNA (rRNA) genes and is separated between the 32 end of 18S rRNA gene and the 52 end of the 5.8S rRNA gene in each transcription unit. The ITS-1 sequences are highly variable between species and are relatively conserved within species. The small subunit ribosomal RNA (SSU rRNA) gene is a well-known marker for molecular characterization. Several studies have addressed the phylogenetic relationships based on 18S rDNA sequences and the morphology of *Eimeria* species, which parasitize domestic fowl (Barta *et al.*, 1997), rodents (Zhao and Duszynski, 2001), rabbits (Kvicerová *et al.*, 2008), cattle (Kokuzawa *et al.*, 2013), goat (Khodakaram *et al.*, 2013), and sheep (Nahavandi *et al.*, 2016). The ITS1 and 18S rDNA gene are useful genetic markers for the specific identification and differentiation of *Eimeria* spp. in ruminants based on this, genetic characterization of the *E. arloingi* in an Iranian native kid have been studied (Khodakaram *et al.*, 2013). Recently in Australia and Myanmar, the use of 18Sr DNA and COI genes for molecular characterization of *Eimeria* species in sheep and goats have been studied ((Al-Habsi *et al.*, 2017; Bawm *et al.*, 2020).

Prevention and Control

Prevention of coccidiosis is preferable to treatment because subclinical production losses and potential permanent damage that is unresponsive to treatment are expensive and have implications for animal welfare. To develop immunity, some exposure to the organism is required, but it should be kept to a minimum. It is critical to reduce stress and other diseases, as well as to improve nutrition and reduce environmental contamination. Overcrowding should be avoided, feed and water should be clean, and daily faeces removal and proper urine drainage are essential. Desiccation and exposure to sunlight are two effective ways to reduce the number of oocysts in the environment. When environmental control is inappropriate, the use of anticoccidial drugs for both treatment and prevention can be advantageous. Anticoccidial medications work by inhibiting the growth and reproduction of coccidian parasites. They have little effect on existing infections, but they should aid in limiting subclinical and clinical disease as well as environmental contamination. Several anticoccidial drugs are available for the treatment and prevention of coccidiosis in ruminants. The most commonly used anticoccidial drugs are ionophores (decoquinate, lasalocid, and monensin) and they are feed additives that are antibiotic-classified. They also improve feed efficiency and control bloat and acidosis by altering the rumen bacteria. Sulfa drugs are commonly used to treat coccidiosis in a variety of species, but the exact mechanism is unknown. Their clinical efficacy may be due to the control of secondary bacterial enteritis rather than a direct effect on coccidia. Sulfaquinoxaline is the only sulfa drug approved for the treatment of coccidiosis in cattle.

Current Status of Anticoccidial Drug Resistance

The World Health Organization Scientific Group (World Health Organization, 1965) developed the definition of resistance in broad terms as 'the ability of a parasite strain to survive and/or to multiply despite the administration and absorption of a drug given in doses equal to or higher than those usually recommended but within the limits of tolerance of the subject'. Such a general definition could be accepted as a basis for the discussions on coccidiosis. Anticoccidial drug resistance mostly reported in poultry while only a few studies have reported in other animals, particularly porcine (Sheresta *et al.*, 2017), ovine (Odden *et al.*, 2018), and caprine *Eimeria* species (Paul and Sharma, 2014; Hsieh *et al.*, 2020). Toltrazuril was the first drug to be shown to reduce efficacy against *Eimeria* species, followed by amprolium.

Evaluation of Anticoccidial Efficacy/Resistance in Ruminants

Long-term anticoccidial drug use is the primary cause of anticoccidial drug resistance (ACR). It has mostly been reported in the poultry industry. Despite the widespread use of anticoccidials in mammals, anticoccidial resistance has only been documented in porcine (Sheresta *et al.*, 2017), ovine (Odden *et al.*, 2018), and caprine *Eimeria* spp (Paul and Sharma, 2014; Hsieh *et al.*, 2020). Testing for anticoccidial efficacy (ACE) in poultry involves the use of histopathological observations and the combination of different indexes, such as oocyst index, body weight gain, relative weight gain, lesion scores, and anticoccidial index (Chapman, 1998). Following are the few methods available for evaluating anticoccidial efficacy in animals.

In vitro Assay for the Evaluation of ACE

In vitro anticoccidial efficacy testing has been widely used in the poultry industry to test both commercial drugs and plant extracts (Alnassan *et al.*, 2015; Thabet *et al.*, 2015; Thabet *et al.*, 2017). In animals, *in vitro* assays have been developed, but they have primarily focused on immunology, parasite-cell interactions, and pathogenicity rather than drug efficacy. The problems in developing such an *in vitro* assay are partly due to the wide size variation among *Eimeria* spp., as purifying oocysts is easier with oocysts of similar size. Furthermore, choosing an infection-friendly cell line is critical because sporozoites must be able to infect and develop in the cells, and the cells must also be able to incorporate the antiococcidial drug.

1. *In vitro* Culture Method or Sporozoite Intracellular Development Assay (SIDA)

Recently, Odden *et al.* (2019) described a sporozoite intracellular development assay (SIDA) to assess the effect of anticoccidials on ovine *Eimeria* species. In this assay, invasion rate and degree of development from sporozoite to both immature and mature schizont are important. The SIDA investigates whether parasites are able to complete their development *in vitro* in the presence of an anticoccidial. In order to perform such an assay, a monolayer of cells must be cultured, and sporozoites from the oocysts must be able to infect and develop in these cells in appropriate conditions. Ruminant *Eimeria* sporozoites are shown to infect a range of cells, such as bovine colonic epithelial cells (BCEC), bovine, human, and caprine umbilical vein endothelial cells (BUVEC, HUVEC, and CUVEC), bovine foetal gastrointestinal cells (BFGC), African green monkey kidney cells (VERO), and Madin-Darby bovine kidney (MDBK). However, further development from sporozoites to schizonts and merozoites is predominantly reported from ruminant intestinal or primary cell lines (Hermosilla *et al.*, 2002; Ruiz *et al.*, 2010; Hermosilla *et al.*, 2015; Carrau *et al.*, 2016). The main limitation of this assay is the purification of oocysts, which is primarily due to the large variation in size between *Eimeria* species with either smaller, larger, or both oocysts being lost in the process. Isolating oocysts, sporulating and excystation of sporulated oocysts, and collecting sporozoites are all part of this assay. Excystation is accomplished using cysteine digestion, followed by digestion in a solution containing a combination of Hank's balanced salt solution, trypsin, and bile (Fayer and Hammond 1967; Pérez *et al.*, 2015). Free sporozoites infected a monolayer of bovine colonic epithelial cells (BCEC), with continuous inclusion of an anticoccidial drug. The invasion rate is determined 24 hours after infection, and intracellular development is evaluated at 8 and 15 days post infection. At day 8 after infection, the number of immature schizonts is evaluated, while at day 15, the number, size and appearance of mature schizonts are assessed. Both commercial anticoccidials (toltrazuril, diclazuril, decoquinate, and sulpha) and pure/derivate anticoccidials (pure toltrazuril,

toltrazuril sulphone, and toltrazuril sulphoxide) are tested in this assay and the parasite development is compared with control cultures to which had been added dimethyl sulphoxide (DMSO) or dimethyl formamide (DMF).

2. Sporozoites Viability Assay

This assay has widely used in the poultry industry to test plant extracts (Cedric *et al.*, 2018). In this test, sporulated oocysts are first isolated, excysted and then the free sporozoites are washed with HBSS and counted in a Malassez counting chamber. A 24-multiwell tissue culture plate is used to evaluate the *in vitro* sporocidal activities. Each well contained a total volume of 2 ml of each concentration of anti coccidial drugs and inoculated with equal number of sporozoites. For comparison, dimethyl sulphoxide (DMSO) or dimethyl formamide (DMF) are used as the reference drug. The set up is examined after 12 h and 24 h. The number of viable and non-viable sporozoites is counted and the percentage of viability is estimated by counting the number of viable sporozoites in a total of 100 sporozoites. The viability inhibitory (Vi) percentage is calculated as follows.

$$\text{Vi per cent} = \frac{\text{Vi per cent of control} - \text{Vi per cent of treated}}{\text{Vi per cent of control}} \times 100$$

3. Oocyst Sporulation Inhibition Assay (OSIA)

The sporulation rate after anticoccidial treatment can be investigated using an oocyst sporulation inhibition assay. Different OSIAs have been used for both avian and animals *Eimeria* species (Saratsis *et al.*, 2012; Habibi *et al.*, 2016). Briefly, 1.5 ml Eppendorf tubes has filled with a 20 µl suspension of 5000 unsporulated oocysts in sterile PBS, 30 µl distilled H_2O, 50 µl of 10 per cent potassium dichromate and 100 µl of different anticoccidials (A-D: 0.5, 0.1, 0.05 and 0.025 mg/ml). The incubations have performed at room temp for 24 h and then the oocysts have washed in distilled water four times (2000×g, 10 min). After the last washing step, the oocysts have resuspended in 1 ml 2 per cent potassium dichromate and transferred into 24-multiwell tissue culture plates and incubated in the presence of oxygen at room temperature. As negative controls, similar concentrations of DMSO or DMF to those used to dissolve the corresponding anticoccidials (from 8 per cent to 1 per cent) has used, and serial formaldehyde solutions served as positive controls (4, 2, 1 and 0.5 per cent). Oocyst sporulation rate will determined after 72 h at room temperature by microscopic analysis, and for this purpose a minimum of 100 oocysts has been counted and analysed.

In vivo Evaluation of ACE

1. Faecal Oocysts Count Reduction Test (FOCRT)

FOCRT is based on the faecal egg count reduction test, with some modifications due to significant biological differences between *Eimeria* and helminths, specifically differences in *Eimeria* oocyst and helminth egg excretion (Chapman, 1974; Sréter *et al.*, 1994; Zaros *et al.*, 2014). The FOCRT is to determine the timing of treatment and sampling, which is based on the increase in oocyst excretion in the control animals. However, due to the wide range of oocyst excretion, statistically significant differences may be difficult to detect.

2. Controlled Efficacy Trial

Randomized controlled trials are widely considered the gold standard for determining drug efficacy. CETs have been performed for the evaluation/verification of drug efficacy/resistance in ruminant helminths (De Graef *et al.*, 2012; Peña-Espinoza *et al.*, 2014). A CET is performed by infecting animals with a suspected resistant isolate; animals are then treated and subsequently euthanized for analysis of parasite burden, a procedure not applicable for routine diagnosis. 20-30 young animals raised protected against exposure to coccidia, are infected with a field isolate of 100,000 *Eimeria* spp. oocysts. At day 7 post-infection, half of the animals are orally treated with 20 mg/kg Toltrazuril or other anticoccidial drugs while the other animals (controls) are given physiological saline. Clinical examinations are conducted, and weight gains recorded. Daily faecal samples are scored for diarrhoea on a scale from 1 to 5, and oocyst excretion is determined using a modified McMaster technique. Oocysts are morphologically identified to species level. At 17–24 days post-infection, the animals are euthanized and necropsied.

Control Strategies

Anticoccidial drug resistance has been reported in ruminant *Eimeria* species, indicating that resistance is possible, as with poultry coccidiosis. Therefore, alternative treatment strategies and management practices must be prioritized in order to maintain productivity and animal welfare. Although good husbandry can help reduce the risk of coccidiosis-causing parasite transmission, more measures are required to totally eliminate the disease.

Management

Hygiene

Hygiene is vital to reducing infection pressure both indoors and on pasture (Taylor, 2000), and faecal contamination of food and water should be avoided, for example, by raising the height of food and water troughs (Daugschies and Najdrowski, 2005). Since oocysts are excreted with faeces, removing faeces through thorough cleaning and drying would significantly reduce the infection pressure of ruminant *Eimeria* species (Ernst *et al.*, 1985; Daugschies and Najdrowski, 2005). However, the use of chemical compounds after cleaning may be impractical for routine use in animal production, but it could serve as an alternative/supplement to reduce infection pressures in highly contaminated facilities.

Grazing Strategies

Ruminant *Eimeria* oocysts can survive on pasture for at least a year (Helle, 1970; Svensson, 1995; Lassen *et al.*, 2013). Pastures that have previously been grazed by young animals are thus considered contaminated and a major source of infection for susceptible animals. Due to *Eimeria* species have host-specific characteristics, rotational grazing or co-grazing with other livestock, as has been observed with helminths, may also reduce the risk of infection (Waller, 2006). It has also been shown that cattle farms that kept sheep on the same pastures as their cattle had a lower likelihood of *Eimeria* spp. positive faecal samples in their cattle (Mitchell *et al.*, 2012).

Nutritional Supplementation

Mineral and vitamin supplementation to young animals can reduce the ingestion, subsequent excretion of *Eimeria* oocysts, and thereby decrease reliance on anticoccidial drugs. Mineral and vitamins is an important component or cofactor in many proteins and enzymes, such as haemoglobin and myoglobin (Weiss, 2010). Housed lambs often are iron deficient (Green *et al.*, 1993; Vatn and Framstad, 2000; Radostits *et al.*, 2007b), and iron deficiency anaemia may lead to abnormal appetite and pica, *i.e.* ingestion of material other than food, including soil (Radostits *et al.*, 2007), and thus, may cause excessive uptake of *Eimeria* oocysts.

Trickle Infections

While *E. crandallis* and *E. ovinoidalis* are highly pathogenic to naive lambs when infected at 4-5 weeks of age, lambs are resistant to infection when infected within the first 72 hours of life (Gregory *et al.*, 1989). It has also been demonstrated that repeated low doses of pathogenic *Eimeria* spp., also known as trickle infection, can induce protective immunity (Catchpole and Gregory, 1985; Gregory *et al.*, 1989). However, under natural conditions, trickle infections are both impractical and nearly impossible to control (Catchpole *et al.*, 1993; Gregory, 1995).

Use of Bioactive Substance and Herbal Extract

Different bioactive substances and extracts from various plant species have been investigated for anticoccidial activities in different hosts, both in vivo and in vitro, including: sainfoin (*Onobrychis viciifolia*), carob pods (*Ceratonia siliqua*), pomegranate (*Punica granatum*) peel extract, grape seed proanthocyanidin extracts (GSPE), and antioxidants such as artemisinin (*Artemisia annua*) (Allen *et al.*, 1998; Naidoo *et al.*, 2008; Wang *et al.*, 2008; Dkhil, 2013; Saratsis *et al.*, 2016). However, none of these bioactive substances have yet to be commercialised for the prevention or control of clinical coccidiosis.

Chapter 22

Anticocccidial Drug Resistance in Poultry and its Mitigation Strategies

R. Garg

Division of Parasitology,
ICAR-Indian Veterinary Research Institute,
Izatnagar, Bareilly – 243122, Uttar Pradesh

Introduction

Coccidiosis, caused by enteric protozoan parasites belonging to the genus *Eimeria,* is one of the most important impediments in raising poultry profitably throughout the world as it causes high morbidity, mortality, poor performance in infected birds. Poultry coccidiosis has been ranked in the top three diseases of poultry in the United Kingdom (UK) based on economic significance, and in the top ten veterinary diseases based on impact on the poor in South Asia. In a 2019 survey of broiler veterinarians in the United States (US), coccidiosis (specifically *Eimeria maxima*) was ranked as the top disease-related issue. Globally, poultry coccidiosis results in economic losses to the tune of approximately £10.4 billion. The estimated annual loss to the Indian poultry industry due to coccidiosis is approximately £447.01 million.

Due to the ubiquitous and fecund nature of the parasite, finding a commercial flock that is not shedding eimerian oocysts is rare. In such a scenario, control of chicken coccidiosis in commercial flocks is of paramount importance. Control of coccidiosis can be achieved either by the inclusion of drugs in the feed or water (prophylactic chemotherapy) or by vaccination. Prophylaxis has been the preferred method for the control of coccidiosis in poultry because once clinical signs become apparent, it is often too late to prevent the pathological consequences of infection. The concept of coccidiosis prevention in chickens by inclusion of drugs in the feed (chemoprophylaxis) was first described in 1948 and involved the use of sulfaquinoxaline, the first feed additive for poultry. In the years that followed, many other drugs were introduced, and until the introduction of ionophores in the 1970s, chemoprophylactic control of coccidiosis was based on the use of such synthetic anticoccidials. Diclazuril was the last anticoccidial drug to be introduced in 1990, and unfortunately, no new drugs in either category have been approved for use for decades. However, the use of anticoccidials as feed additives is posing a problem to the poultry industry due to development of drug resistance, changing consumer values and growing awareness about the drug and chemical residues in meat and eggs.

The current approach to delay the onset of resistance is to employ rotation programs combined with good husbandry, chemoprophylaxis, and/or live parasite vaccination. However, for the control of coccidiosis in the future, novel cost-effective preventative chemotherapy, subunit or recombinant vaccines or alternate parasite control strategies are desperately needed.

Anticoccidial Drugs

Anticoccidial drugs fall into two categories, the synthetic compounds (produced by chemical synthesis and popularly known as 'chemicals') and the ionophore antibiotics, which are by-products of bacterial fermentation. Synthetic drugs were the first to be discovered and comprise a diverse array of molecules that are absorbed into the blood stream of the host and kill developing parasites in epithelial cells of villi in the intestine. Ionophores have a different mode of action from synthetic drugs since they are able to destroy motile stages of the *Eimeria* life cycle (sporozoites and merozoites) in the gut lumen or following cell penetration. Since the introduction of monensin in 1972, ionophores have been the most widely used anticoccidial drugs for the control of coccidiosis. Table 22.1 enlists the anticoccidial drugs commonly used in poultry industry along with their mode of action.

Table 22.1: Common Anticoccidial Drugs with their Mode of Action

Anticoccidial Drug	*Mode of Action*	*Affected Life Cycle Stages*
Sulfonamides	Inhibition of folic acid pathway	2ndand later schizonts
Amprolium	Thiamine antagonist	2ndgeneration schizont
Decoquinate	Inhibit respiration by blocking electron transport in parasite mitochondrion	Sporozoite
Clopidol	Affects electron transport	Sporozoite
Benzeneamines	Uncouple oxidative phosphorylation	Sporozoites
Monensin	Influx of sodium ions	Sporozoite

Anticoccidial Drug	Mode of Action	Affected Life Cycle Stages
Robenidine	Bind to proteins and cause uncoupling of parasite mitochondria	Multiple stages
Halofuginone	Unknown	Asexual stages
Ionophores	Cation transport across cell membrane	Sporozoites and merozoites
Diclazuril	Nucleotide analogue	Sexual and asexual stages
Toltrazuril	Act against plastid like genome	Multiple stages

Anticoccidial Drug Resistance

The development of drug resistance in *Eimeria* is common because of extensive use of anticoccidial drugs for the control of avian coccidiosis. In 1965, the World Health Organization Scientific Group defined resistance as "the ability of a parasite strain to survive and/or to multiply despite the administration and absorption of a drug given in doses equal to or higher than those usually recommended but within the limits of tolerance of the subject". Drug resistance is a genetic phenomenon, and once established in a line of coccidian, it remains for many years. Different types of anticoccial drug resistance are described below:

Acquired Resistance

When resistance results from heritable decrease in sensitivity of certain strains and species of *Eimeria* to the drugs with the passage of time, it is termed as acquired resistance. Depending on the extent of sensitivity of the drug lost, it may be partial or complete. Further, there is a direct relationship between concentration of the drug and degree of resistance. The use of lower concentration of a drug below recommended levels allows for the selection of resistant mutants over a period of time. Most of the sulphonamides and polyether ionophores develop this type of resistance if not used judiciously.

Cross Resistance

Cross-resistance is the sharing of resistance among different compounds with a similar mode of action. A high degree of cross resistance has been reported among maduramicin, monensin, salinomycin, narasin, and lasalocid. However, this may not always occur as a number of reports are available stating that maduramicin was effective in controlling isolates of *Eimeria* resistant to other ionophores. In general, it is advised that, if the routinely used anticoccidial is ineffective, it is preferable to use other anticoccidial that does not share a similar mode of action.

Multiple Resistance

Multiple resistance is a resistance to more than one drug, even though they have different modes of action. There may be many reasons for the development of multiple resistance in field isolates of *Eimeria* strains *viz.* sequential exposure to the compounds in question in successive flocks or genetic recombination between different *Eimeria* strains that are exposed to different anticoccidials.

Emergence and spread of resistance is very rapid in case of field isolates of *Eimeria*. A number of factors may be involved in the development of anticoccidial resistance which include:

- ✰ Parasite genetic factors that are not under human control *viz.* dominance of resistant alleles, number of genes involved, initial frequency of resistance genes, genetic diversity of population, relative fitness of resistant organisms, chance of linkage disequilibrium and opportunity for genetic recombination.
- ✰ Factor related to type of anticoccidial used and it's application *viz.* chemical nature of drug, drug persistence in the host, drug clearance kinetics, selection threshold, life stage(s) targeted, mode of application, frequency of treatment, timing of treatments, spatial use of treatments, under-dosing *etc.*
- ✰ Biological factors *viz.* biotic factors like generation time, offspring per generation and breeding patterns, and behavioural factors that affect gene flow and the chance of selection like isolation, mobility, migration, monophagy or polyphagy, fortuitous survival and refugia.

A number of mechanisms are known by which coccidia become resistant to anticoccidial drugs. This may involve altered permeability of the cell membrane so that the drug is no longer taken up or is rapidly pumped out of the cell (ionophores), inhibiting/blocking the biochemical pathway and/or use of an alternative biochemical pathway (sulpha drugs, clopidol, quinolones), and modification of the target sites in the coccidia parasites (amprolium).

Detection of Anticoccidial Drug Resistance

Several indices are used to evaluate the efficacy of anticoccidial drugs. These indices use several factors like weight gain, feed conversion ratio, lesion score, oocyst output, survival rate *etc.* Understanding of these factors is fundamental to evaluate the wide spread development of resistance using various indices. The following indices are used to detect anticoccidial drug resistance:

Global Index (GI)

GI is calculated on the basis of weight gain (per cent), feed conversion (g/g), lesion scores, oocyst index and mortality (per cent) by using the following formula:

GI= per cent WGNNC–[(FM–FNNC)×10]–(OIM – OIINC)–[(LSM – LSINC)×2]–(per cent mortality/2), Where WG: weight gain, F: Feed conversion ratio, WG: Weight gain, F: Feed conversion ratio, OI: Oocyst index, LS: Lesion score, M: Medicated group, NNC: Non infected Non medicated control group, INC: Infected non-medicated control group.

Drugs with global index of ≥90 per cent are considered highly effective and those having global index of <50 per cent indicate resistance.

Anticoccidial Sensitivity Test (AST)

It is calculated based on the reduction of mean lesion score of the treatment group compared with the infected non-medicated group. Mean lesion score reduction of 0-30 per cent indicate resistance and more than 50 per cent reduction indicate full sensitivity.

Optimum Anticoccidial Activity (OAA)

In this index, a growth and survival ratio (GSR) is used to calculate the percentage of OAA. Value of ≤50 per cent indicate resistance and ≥75 per cent indicate sensitivity.

Anticoccidial Index (ACI)

ACI is calculated on the basis of relative weight gain (per cent), survival rate (per cent), lesion score value and oocyst score by using the following formula:

ACI= (Relative weight gain rate+survival rate) - (Lesion scorex 10+oocyst value/score).

ACI value of 180 or higher indicate that drug is very effective and value <120 indicate that the drug is not effective.

Anticoccidial Drug Resistance In India

Anticoccidial drug resistance was first recorded against sulphaquinoxaline in *Eimeria tenella* from USA in the year 1954. Since then, resistance to almost all anticoccidials used in poulty industry has been reported from various parts of the world. Anticoccidial drug resistance in India was first reported by Panda *et al.*(1973). They found that when bifuran and sulphaquinoxaline were given continuously for3 years, their efficacy against *Eimeria* sp. got reduced due to development of resistants trains. Later, Gill and Bajwa (1979) from Punjab (north India) reported the resistanceof sulfaquinoxaline, nitrofurazone plus furazolidone, amprolium, clopidol and nicarbazinin various field isolates of *Eimeria* sp. Rana (1993) found resistance in *E. tenella* against clopidol and nitrofurazone plus furazolidone and sodium sulphadimethyl pyrimidine in Haryana. Yadav and Gupta (2001) reported partial resistance against Salinomycin in an *E. tenella* isolate from Haryana. Later, limited efficacy of monensin in a field isolate of *E. tenella* from Jind district of Haryana was reported by Gautam and Gupta (2004). Lately, Agarwal *et al.* (2013) reported resistance against clopidol, meduramicin and diclazuril in some isolates of *E. tenella* infecting chickens from Hisar, Haryana.

Mitigation Stratagies for Control of Anticoccidial Resistance

Various approaches for management and control of anticoccidial drug resistance are described below:

- ☆ ***Biosecurity measures*:** Biosecurity may help to reduce contamination between many facets of the poultry industry. Proper biosecurity measures help to reduce the risk of contamination among birds or from pests (*e.g.* vermin or flying insects) in a single flock or between flocks due to carryover of used litter or an improperly cleaned poultry house. To prevent the introduction of *Eimeria* sp. to the farm the biosecurity measures should focus on: separation of the farm by fencing, and other animals including rodents and insects should be kept out; entry should be restricted at the farm and traffic between farms should be restricted; and strict sanitation including disinfection of materials, people and equipment entering the farm and poultry house. Care takers should change the complete dress before visiting the new poultry house to minimize the spread of eimerian oocysts.
- ☆ ***Managemental practices:*** The main factors of consideration in the environmental management are good ventilation, thorough clean out between flocks, removal of moisture sources and keeping the litter dry, optimum bird density, low stress and good feed and water management. Leaving the shed empty for a period between flocks will allow the destruction of oocysts. Caretakers should change the complete dress before visiting the new poultry house to minimise the spread of resistant oocysts. Keeping the older birds away from chicks will prevent build-up of infection in the farm as old birds are carriers of coccidial infection.
- ☆ ***Regular monitoring for drug resistance:*** In order to reduce the development of resistance, knowledge of the *Eimeria* species present and resistance status should be determined before the selection of anticoccidial drugs. Unfortunately, tools to determine resistance status rapidly are not available. Development of *in vitro* tests for this purpose would be very useful. The development of mathematical models to help understand coccidia dynamics, drug resistance and production systems would be a valuable advancement.
- ☆ ***Introducing shuttle and/or rotational programmes:*** In *Shuttle programme,* two or more drugs belonging to different classes of anticoccidials are used within a single flock *e.g.,* use of one class of drug in starter feed, another in growers, returning to the first for the finisher diet, followed by a withdrawal diet. The short period of use of each class probably provides insurance against one drug class failing.

  In *Bio-Shuttle programme,* anticoccidial vaccines and drugs are administered alternatively during different age groups of birds. On day 1, anticoccidial vaccine is administered, on day 14-28 anticoccidial drug is given in grower feed, and on day 28-38, the same anticoccidial drug or a different anticoccidial drug in finisher feed at low dose is administered. For example, Advent® which is a live vaccine containing oocysts of *E. tenella*, *E. maxima* and *E. acervulina* is administered on day 1 followed by Salinomycin (60 g/ton) on day 14-28 and Lincomycin (4 g/ton) on day 28-38. Results revealed improvement in feed conversion ratio and an increase in body weight gain of birds.

In *Rotational programme*, drug classes are rotated from one batch to another, not within a single batch. Such programmes may also be chosen for its convenience in feed mills rather than as a scientifically based method for reducing selection for resistance.

In *'Step down' programme*, the concentrations of the anticoccidial drugs are reduced as the birds get older. This may be helpful in the development of immunity in the older birds, but on the other hand, this practice can cause selection for drug resistance.

- ***Restoration of drug sensitivity by introducing drug sensitive coccidia:*** The pattern of drug sensitivity in a population of coccidia can be greatly altered by the introduction of drug-sensitive coccidia, which can be accomplished through the use of non-attenuated coccidiosis vaccines, use of drug-sensitive laboratory-maintained lines and admixture of sensitive and resistant strains and propagating in unmedicated chicken.

- ***Use of botanical/herbal anticoccidials/natural products:*** Although chemoprophylaxis is cost-effective and largely successful for control of coccidiosis, the presence of drug resistance and public demands for residue-free meat has encouraged development of alternative control strategies, most of which are natural compounds extracted from plants or produced by microorganisms. Some of these compounds are antioxidants that damage the parasite, thus preventing the infection. Others, such as essential oils, disrupt the structure of oocysts preventing the dispersion of the parasite. The immunoactive components of some of the plants and fungi include polysaccharides, glycosides, alkaloids, volatile oils, and organic acids, of which polysaccharides are considered to be the most important. Polysaccharides may act as immune enhancers or immunomodulators. Extracts of *Sophora flavescens Aiton* was the most effective in reducing lesion scores, maintaining body weight gain, and reducing oocyst production. Use of mushroom polysaccharides has also been found to be effective. A number of plant products are commercially available on the market and they can be used as anticoccidial feed additives in chickens and/or other animals, like Cocci-Guard (DPI Global, USA), a mixture of *Quercus infectoria*, *Rhus chinensis*, and *Terminalia chebula* (Kemin Industries, USA), Apacox (GreenVet, Italy), BP formulation made up of *Bidens pilosa* and other plants (Ta-Fong Inc., Taiwan),Zycox containing *Hobrrhena antidysentrica*, *Berberis aristata*, *Embelia ribes* and *Acorus calamus etc.* These herbal anticoccidials cause least interference to the natural development of immunity, are safe, not likely to induce drug resistance and are friendly to the environment, producers, and consumers.

- ☆ ***Use of Probiotics and other feed aditives:*** Probiotics modify receptors on enterocytes. This impairs or destroys sporozoites/and or merozoites from penetrating an enterocyte. This is usually used in combination with vaccines. *Lactobacillus, Enterococcus, Pediococcus* and *Bacillus, Saccharomyces cerevisiae, Enterococcus faecium* are some of the bacteria used as probiotics. Sources of fats containing high concentrations of n-3 fatty acids (n-3 FA) (docosahexaenoic acid, eicosapentaenoic acid, linolenic acid), such as fish oils, flaxseed oil, and whole flaxseed, Vitamin A, Betaine, CpG oligodeoxynucleotides (ODNs) are also feed additives found beneficial in coccidiosis. Direct fed microbials (DFM; *Aspergillus oryzae* and *Bacillus subtilis*) have also been found to be useful.
- ☆ ***Anticoccidial vaccines:*** The emergence of multi-drug resistant strains and growing concerns of drug residues warrants for the development of an effective vaccine against the disease. Currently available vaccines against poultry coccidiosis are mostly based upon varied formulations of live virulent or attenuated parasites. Commercially available anticoccidial vaccines include Advent, Coccivac-B, Coccivac-D, Coccivac-T, *Eimeria*vax 4M, Inovocox, Immucox I, Immucox II, Immucox T, Hatchpak Cocci III, Paracox 5, Paracox 8, Livacox Q, Livacox T and Hipracox *etc.* The production of live vaccines is limited by low reproductive index of the parasite and high production costs, among other factors. Immune stimulating antigens having defined roles in parasite invasion, establishment and multiplication can be potential vaccine candidates and pave way for development of subunit vaccines against coccidiosis. Of late, a subunit vaccine named 'CoxAbic®', which is based on affinity purified gametocyte antigen of *E. maxima* has been marketed in Israel. A number of novel antigens that could be used to generate potent recombinant anticoccidial vaccines have been identified including, MICs (MIC1 to MIC5), AMA1, IMP1, LDH, SO7, SAG, Em14-3-3, T4A, Profilin, Rhomboid associate protein, ROPJ, Gametocyte antigens *viz.* Gam86, Gam56, Gam22 *etc.* Cocktail immunization with different recombinant proteins as well as other putative vaccine candidates of *Eimeria,* targeting different life cycle stages of the parasite can further strengthen the endeavor of recombinant antigen based vaccine for poultry coccidiosis.
- ☆ ***Improving genetic resistance in birds:*** Different strains of domestic poultry have been assessed for their capability to resist coccidial infections. The importance of the host genetics on the outcome of thedisease has been demonstrated by comparisons of inbred lines or more infrequently of outbred lines.

- ☆ ***Use of nanotechnology for improving delivery of anticoccidials:*** Nanoparticles are a recent trend and when supplemented in abird's diet are called as "nanobiotics". Silver nanoparticles have been used as an additive in poultry feeds as coccidiostat and have shown to reduce *E. tenella* oocyst output by 50 per cent. For broiler chickens, nanoparticles of selenium are a highly bioavailable and non-toxic alternative as it increased absorption and diffusion of materials into organs and tissues, and increased antioxidant capacity. Atoltrazuril mixed nanomicelle (TMNM) delivery system was developed that significantly increases in the drugs olubility and bioavailability.

Conclusions

To date coccidiosis control has relied mainly on chemoprophylaxis, however, the occurrence of drug resistance and the increasing concerns among consumers has led to the quest for alternative control strategies. Regular monitoring of *Eimeria* species for development of resistance against different anticoccidial groups has a crucial role in the management of resistance and for making a correct choice of an effective drug. Success in management of anticoccidial drug resistance depends on an integrated approach involving management, judicious use of existing anticoccidials, immunological control measures and alternate "drug-free" strategies. Educating the farmers about recommended coccidiosis control practices as strategic and/or tactic measures would be rewarding.

Chapter 23

Nutritional Management to Reduce the Risk of Anti-parasitic Drug Resistance in Livestock

M.K. Mehta[1] *and V. Agrawal*

[1]*Dean Faculty,*
Nanaji Deshmukh Veterinary Science University (NDVSU),
Jabalpur – 482004, Madhya Pradesh
Assistant Professor, Department of Veterinary Parasitology,
College of Veterinary Science and Animal Husbandry NDVSU,
Jabalpur – 453446, Madhya Pradesh

Introduction

There are a variety of internal and external factors that influence animal production performance, with parasites and parasitism being one of the most significant restrictions to animal output, particularly in tropical nations. Because of the rising development of resistance to these compounds, the traditional mode of control of these gastro-intestinal parasites (GIP) based on the repeated administration of anthelmintics is now seriously questioned. Among the currently known alternatives to anthelmintics, manipulating host nutrition to promote host resistance and/or resilience to parasite infections appears to be one of the most promising strategies for reducing reliance on conventional chemotherapy and favoring long-term GIP control. Feed intake and nutrient requirements have long been recognised as essential factors in influencing animal production efficiency. Parasites and parasitism are substantial restrictions to animal output, especially in tropical countries. The gastro-intestinal (GI) nematode causes the majority of parasite infections in domestic animals. This can lead to appetite loss, impaired Gl functioning, changes in protein, energy, and mineral metabolism, and alterations in water balance. The ability of the host to cope with the repercussions of parasitism, as well as to contain and eventually conquer parasitism, is influenced by nutrition. Since it is hypothesized that the host prioritizes the reversal of parasitic patho-physiological consequences over other body functions, improved nutrition should always result in improved parasitism reversal. The relationships between nutrition and parasitism will be discussed, which will include both quantitative (impact of protein, energy, micronutrients, and other phyto-additives) and qualitative (organic livestock farming, foraging) components of the diet. Nutrition's beneficial effects, particularly the necessity of protein nutrition in maintaining parasite immunity, the potential use of innovative crops, and biological control options have all been studied. Biological control of nematodes appears to have a bright future, however in order to help farmers, the best delivery mechanism must be modified and improved. Furthermore, more work will be required to identify anthelmintic resistance, non-chemical alternatives to parasite management, modification of parasite immunity by genetic and nutritional factors, an integrated parasite control approach, and the appropriate application of these technologies in various geographic regions. Internal parasites pose a severe threat to the health, welfare, and productivity of organically managed cattle. While the ultimate goal is to eliminate antiparasitic drug use, this is rarely achieved in practice. It is now recognized that chemical anthelmintic treatment alone may not be sufficient for long-term parasite management in grazing ruminants.

Managing Parasitism through Nutrition

i. Increasing Feed and Nutrient Consumption

One of the most fundamental aspects that influences the nutritional condition and health of animals is a sufficient level of nutrition. With increasing food intake and body weight, the animals gradually recover. Because of their typical immunocompetence mechanism, the animals eventually appear to be normal. As a direct consequence, palatable feed ingredients or appetite enhancers (micronutrients, processed feed ingredients, flavours, colours, and so on) should be used to restore VFI in parasitized animals, as well as the inclusion of concentrated nutrients (energy and protein) in the feed consumed by animals to meet the minimum maintenance needs during the disease process.

ii. Modulation of the Animal's Immunity through Nutrition

Nutritional modulation of the animal's immunity to infection is one of the most recent methods for parasitic illness control and prevention. The parasite's establishment, development, survival, and fecundity are all affected by acquired immunity in the host (Quinnell and Keymer, 1990). The time it takes for the immune system to recognise the parasite and undergo the alterations that lead to a successful immunological response can range from a few days in protozoan infection to several weeks in helminth infection. The host's diet may have an impact on how quickly immunity is acquired and manifested in response to the parasitism. Changes in nutrient intake are unlikely to alter the early pace of parasite immunity acquisition in young animals under normal nutritional conditions (Coop *et al.*, 1995). The acquisition of immunity is greatly hampered in extremely malnourished animals that lose protein mass. Within the same breed and between breeds with a strong genetic base, there is a lot of inter-animal variance in the pace of resistance development. In cattle (Mausour *et al.*, 1992), sheep (Mausour *et al.*, 1992), and goats (Mausour *et al.*, 1992), host protein and energy nutrition can have a significant impact on the expression of immunity (Coop *et al.*, 1995). Because many components of the immune system's effector arm, such as immunoglobulins, mucoproteins, and cellular products (leukotrienes), are proteinaceous, they are expected to use protein resources in both quantitative and qualitative terms (Yu *et al.*, 1999).

iii. Mineral and Vitamin Supplementation

Mineral and vitamin supplementation can have a big impact on ruminant susceptibility. According to studies on the association between phosphorus (P) and *T. vitrinus* worm burden in sheep, greater P availability reduces mean worm burden (Coop and Field, 1983). Cu, Mo, and Se are known to influence host resistance to nematode infection, possibly through a direct anthelmintic effect, as well as by modulating host metabolism (Coop and Kyriarakis, 1999). Increased levels of selenium and vitamin E were reported to lessen the severity of primary infection and improve weight gain and feed conversion in caecal coccidiosis (*E. tenella*) (Nockels. 1991). The vitamins A, D, and B complex are essential for parasite immunity development. Cobalt is used to manufacture vitamin B12, while iron is an essential mineral. It was also discovered that when the phosphorus content in the meal was 0.28 percent phosphorus on a dry matter basis, the weight growth of parasitized lambs increased by 40 per cent compared to lambs fed a low (0.18 percent) phosphorus diet.

iv. Use of Copper Oxide Wire Particles (CWOP)

COWP treatment appears to have the potential to reduce *Haemonchus* spp. establishment and worm fecundity for an extended period of time, and may provide livestock producers with an additional means of reducing larval contamination of pasture, especially in areas where anthelmintic resistance is a problem and copper supplementation is likely to be beneficial (Knox, 2002). With the lowest concentration of copper in the liver, 2g of COWP was efficient in easing *H. contortus* infection and reducing the quantity of egg-laying nematodes in the abomasum (Burke *et al.*, 2004). Burke and Miller (2006) also discovered that numerous doses of COWP were just as effective as levamisole in controlling *H. contortus* without the risk of copper toxicity. Martinez Ortiz de Montellano *et al.* (2007) found that browsing goats treated with copper oxide needles had lower worm burdens of *H. contortus* and *T. colubriformis* (Copinox. 2 g capsules).

v. Anti-parasitic Herbal Feed Additives

Herbs have been used to treat parasitism and increase cattle performance for years by farmers and traditional healers, and many current commercial treatments are derived from plants. Despite their widespread ethnoveterinary use, scientific evidence on the anti parasite efficacy of most plant products is scarce. Plant secondary metabolites (PSM) as additives in livestock rationing may also have antioxidant and antihelminthic properties, as well as complex formation between protein and condensed tannins, which protects dietary protein from degradation by the symbiotic microflora of foregut fermenters, thereby increasing the animal's use of it. This protein impact is likely to benefit animals only in a limited number of nutrient-rich environments, such as those present in agricultural systems. Plant therapies have been proven in vivo controlled investigations to result in parasitism reductions that are significantly lower than those seen with anthelmintic medications. Plant enzymes, such as cysteine proteinases, or secondary metabolites, such as alkaloids, glycosides, and tannins, have exhibited dose-dependent anti-parasitic activities, despite the fact that the active chemicals in herbal treatments are often unknown. However, because some of the beneficial chemicals may have anti-nutritional consequences, such as lower feed intake and performance, it is critical to establish a link between the anti-parasitic actions of plant products and their anti-nutritional and other side effects.

vi. Use of Condensed Tannin as Anthelmintic

Condensed tannins (CT) have biological effects that may aid in the management of dewormer-resistant internal parasites (IP), hence CT in forages could be used in IP control programmes (Hoste *et al.*, 2005). Plant CT may affect IP in a direct or indirect manner. Direct effects on IP's physiological functioning could be mediated by CT-nematode interactions. By binding to plant proteins in the rumen and limiting microbial breakdown, CT can indirectly improve protein nutrition by increasing amino acid flow to the duodenum. Improved protein feeding has been proven to lower parasite infection in a variety of ovine species. This is thought to be due to increased host immunity. Condensed tannin (CT) supplementation at a moderate dose (1-2 percent of DMI) was found to be beneficial in inhibiting the development of internal parasites and reducing their numbers. Low to moderate CT supplementation increased nutrition consumption, growth performance, and immune responses. As a result, CT supplementation in animal diets acts as a natural dewormer and a sustainable, environmentally and eco-friendly alternative strategy to controlling internal parasites and maintaining normal health, performance, and organic food production for customers.

Maximize Drug Availability and Efficacy by using Host Physiology

Anthelmintic efficacy is proportional to the length of time the medicine is in contact with the parasite. When all other conditions remain constant, the efficacy of many anthelmintics can be enhanced by simply increasing the contact time. As a result, understanding the physiology of the host can be exploited to improve therapeutic efficacy. When treating a ruminant orally, it's vital that the entire dose reaches the rumen. The duration of drug availability in the rumen as it is absorbed from the rumen and moves to more distal sites of absorption is largely determined by the digesta flow rate. Because rumen volume remains relatively constant, feed intake and digesta residence time have an inverse relationship. Simply limiting feed intake for 24 hours before treatment reduces digesta transit and boosts medication availability and efficacy. This impact has been proven in both pharmacokinetic investigations and field efficacy trials, where this method dramatically improved fenbendazole efficacy against benzimidazole field-resistant strains of GI worms. While using a BZ medication, withholding feed is always a good idea, and it's even good when administering Ivermectin. It is not required to restrict feed when using moxidectin or levamisole because an increase in efficacy is unlikely. It's also crucial to use proper technique while drenching animals. Orally administered anthelmintics should be placed over the back of the tongue. Drenching the buccal cavity rather than the pharynx/esophagus can encourage esophageal groove closure with a considerable drench bypassing the rumen. Absorbed drug concentrations may be higher at first, but they are only there for a short time, reducing efficacy. These two recommendations, which require no additional cost or effort, have the potential to considerably improve drug efficacy and hence extend the useful life of today's anthelmintics, and should be employed as a matter of course.

Biological Control

The most viable solution appears to be *Duddingtonia flagrans*, a net-trapping, nematode-destroying fungus. This fungus, which produces a sticky three-dimensional network and has been isolated all over the world, is unique because it can produce large numbers of thick-walled resting spores called chlamydospores, which survive passage through the gastro-intestinal tract of grazing livestock and can grow and trap nematodes, including parasitic nematode larvae. Numerous trials with cattle, sheep, horses, and pigs have proved the fungus's considerable potential as a biological control agent. Despite the fact that the potential utility of *D. flagrans* chlamydospores has been confirmed through several studies, realistic delivery systems such as slow release devices, feed-blocks, or similar are required to effectively exploit this tool in future integrated management approaches. Microfungi for biological control could be introduced as part of a feed supplement or put into feed-blocks for animals reared under relatively intensive conditions.

Conclusion

When anthelmintic are used at high levels, with increasing frequency and improper doses, drug resistance becomes a major issue in small ruminant husbandry. The shift to organic farming techniques has boosted the demand for chemoprophylaxis alternatives in recent years. Improving host resilience and/or infection resistance through management approaches that include nutrition modification can be one component of an integrated approach. The impact of changes in host resistance on host production as a function of nutritional condition needs to be better understood. If producers intend to make stronger use of host acquired immunity and reduce reliance on pesticides for prophylaxis, they must first understand the function of diet in strengthening both resistance and resilience of the host to GI parasites. As a result, future strategies should focus on systematic studies to establish regulatory mechanisms through which therapeutic diets aimed at improving host nutrition while keeping the nutrition-parasitism interrelationship in mind, the role of amino acids, vitamins, and micro nutrients in relation to host resilience/resistance and drug-nutrient interactions for increased therapeutic efficacy parasitism.

Chapter 24

Controlling Antiparasitic Drug Resistance in Livestock Animals using Genetic Approach

M.S. Thakur, S. Joshi, V. Khare, Asit Jain and Akansha Singh

Department of Animal Genetics and Breeding, College of Veterinary Science and Animal Husbandry NDVSU, Jabalpur – 482001, Madhya Pradesh

Introduction

The genetic resistance to disease is a result of a complicated collection of signals and responses with which the individual and pathogen interact. In the past decades, genetics has made a considerable contribution in livestock and poultry health sector as well as in disease resistance. However, curation and prevention of all livestock as well as poultry disease could not be done, as in most of the cases disease resistance is governed by a large number of factors along with the gene networks. To lessen the impact of livestock diseases on animal health and profitability, management, feeding, immunisation, culling, therapeutic treatment, stress reduction strategies, and other measures must be combined with genetic approaches. Resistance to drug is one of the significant and emerging problem in most of the infectious and parasitic diseases in livestock and poultry. Until recently, most of the parasitic and infectious diseases are being treated and managed with the use of many drugs, which has led to drug resistance in many livestock infections (McManus *et al.*, 2014). Drug resistance is described as a heritable decrease in a parasite population's susceptibility to a drug's effect. Identification of markers for drug-resistant parasites will provide the understanding of genetic basis of resistance. Studies have facilitated the understanding of origin and spread of resistance, mode of action of drugs and determine whether the resistant phenotype can be manipulated or reversed. Furthermore, if drug resistance could be diagnosed early, parasites resistant to one drug may be eliminated before the resistant genotype took over. Given that most parasite diseases are treated with a very restricted pharmacopoeia, extending the life of existing medications in the face of rising levels of resistance is critical. Breeding for disease resistance has emerged as a serious concern for animal geneticists. Improved animal welfare, higher efficiency and output, and therefore a decreased environmental imprint, reduced reliance on other disease control strategies, and improved public perception are all advantages of successfully raising animal resistance to parasite disease.

Breeding for disease resistance, on the other hand, poses a number of technical difficulties. Furthermore, despite its apparent advantages, its long-term viability is sometimes questioned due to the risk of parasite evolution, and the function of host genetics within integrated disease management systems is frequently ambiguous. Vaccination, culling unhealthy animals, and selecting resistant animals are all examples of disease control measures (*e.g.*, biosecurity, sanitation).

Resistance to internal parasites has been shown to vary genetically in a variety of species, including humans and livestock (Bishop and Morris, 2007). The genetic architecture underpinning such features, on the other hand, is little understood (Kemper *et al.*, 2013). Genetic factors including breed, G-E interactions, heritability and correlations along with the genetic markers and genomic selection, influence the parasitic control. As a result, because the host-parasite interaction happens on multiple levels, the execution of breeding programmes becomes one of the most critical things to consider.

The selection schemes can impart disease resistance or tolerance. "Resistance" refers to the host's ability to resist infection, whereas "tolerance" means that the host is infected by the pathogen but has no clinical symptoms. Prevention from spreading of the disease to other individuals, disease resistance rather than tolerance is an important concept. When the host's resistance to infection is improved genetically, infection transmission is frequently affected. While genetic tolerance enhancement may minimise clinical indications of sickness, it may not prevent infection spread to other animals (Gibson and Bishop, 2005). This review will look into using genetic selection methods to improve animal responsiveness to helminth challenges.

Antiparasitic Resistance

Antiparasitic resistance is a major threat to livestock production systems around the world, and it's also becoming a major issue in parasite care for companion animals. Human soil-transmitted helminths and filaria are also becoming a growing concern. The capacity to use diagnostic tests to discover antiparasitic resistance at an early stage is a crucial part of managing antiparasitic resistance. Diagnostics may play an essential role in determining which medications remain effective in host-parasite systems where resistance is already widespread (Bishop, 2012).

Antiparasitic resistance refers to parasites' genetic ability to withstand the effects of an antiparasitic medicine to which they were previously exposed. When an increasing proportion of a parasite population carries resistance genes, the parasites can survive treatment with an antiparasitic medicine that was previously effective. Apart from India, antiparasitic resistance in livestock species has been a problem in Australia, New Zealand, South Africa, and South America for decades. Antiparasitic resistance has been detected in livestock species in the United States and also India, according to recent scientific findings (Bishop, 2012).

Importance of Refugia in Drug Resistance

The vulnerable parasites die after an animal is treated with an antiparasitic treatment, while the resistant parasites remain to pass on resistance genes to their offspring. If there aren't enough susceptible parasites in the environment or on the animal, the increase in resistant parasites that occurs after treatment won't be diluted. When there aren't enough refugia, this happens. The proportion of the overall parasite population that is not selected for antiparasitic drug therapy, or those parasites that are in "refuge" from the drug, is referred to as "refugia." As a result, these parasites face no selection pressure to evolve resistance. On the farm, Refugia keeps a proportion of vulnerable parasites, which includes:

- Host-based refugia, parasites in untreated animals.
- Environmental refugia, which are eggs and larvae that are already on the pasture when the animals are treated.
- Parasite life cycles that are unaffected by medication therapy, such as some larval stages.
- Maintaining refugia keeps drug-sensitive (susceptible) parasites alive. The presence of certain drug-sensitive parasites in a parasite population reduces (dilutes) the proportion of resistant parasites (Figure 24.1).

Factors Contributing to Antiparasitic Resistance

- Biology, genetics, and pathogenicity of the parasite
- The host animal's immune state.
- Treatment variables such as dosage and dosing frequency.
- Drug characteristics like mode of action and half-life.
- Some cattle management techniques.

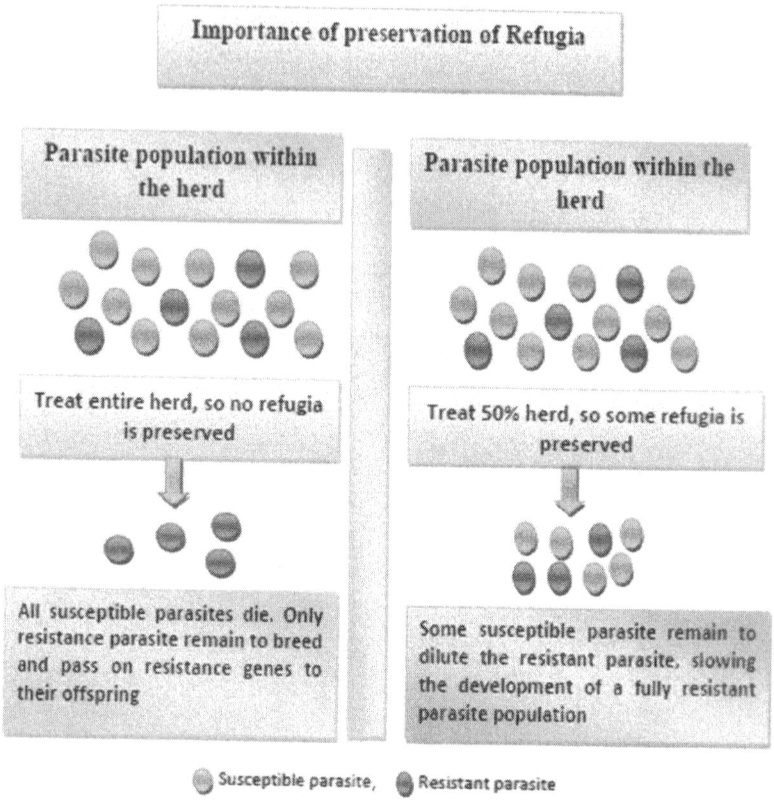

Figure 24.1: Importance of Preservation of Refugia.

Molecular Genetic Approaches for Selection of Disease Resistance

Several biotechnological technologies have been used to transgenically change disease resistance or susceptibility. All genes known to influence non-specific and particular host defence mechanisms against infectious diseases, as well as genes for correcting faulty genes, are targets for gene transfer experiments (Mueller and Brem, 1994). The following are integrated methodologies for identifying the genetics of disease resistance traits shown in Figure 24.2. Animal researchers have benefited greatly from the recent advent of strong statistical tools and computer packages that handle linkage analysis between marker loci and QTL for experimental populations (Cheng *et al.*, 2013). Searching for molecular markers, identifying the underlying genes, construction of linkage maps, *etc.* are the fundamentals for identification of genetic marker. Figure 24.2 illustrates the strategies for disease resistance selection.

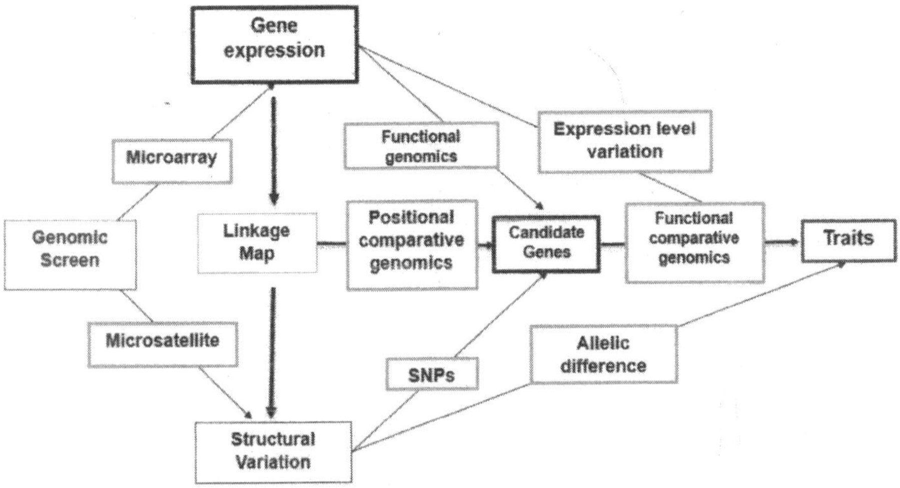

Figure 24.2: Integrated Strategies to Identify Genetics of Disease Resistance Traits.

Relationship of Genes and their Products to Intermediate Phenotypes

Figure 24.3 depicts the interaction between a gene and its product with a single pathway that, when malfunctioned, may lead to disease.

Search for DNA Markers for Resistance

In domesticated animals, the single-locus disorders were among the first Mendelian traits to be identified and to be included in early linkage maps after the rediscovery of Mendelism. The use of linkage maps and comparative genomics has proved critical in identifying the causal gene for single-locus illnesses with significant clinical implications. In domestic animals, the 'score-card' now includes more than 100 disorders for which a molecular lesion has been found and thus a DNA test is accessible. Selection on estimated breeding values for liability could considerably improve the effectiveness of control methods for multifactorial illnesses that are scored on an all-or-none basis or into numerous classes. Selection based on predicted breeding values for liability could considerably improve the effectiveness of control strategies. Resistance to diseases and parasites has a lot of genetic diversity. As a result, resistance selection can be successful. Because of the technical and welfare issues associated with exposing animals to viruses or parasites in order to select for resistance, there is a rapid search for resistance DNA markers (Bishop, 2012).

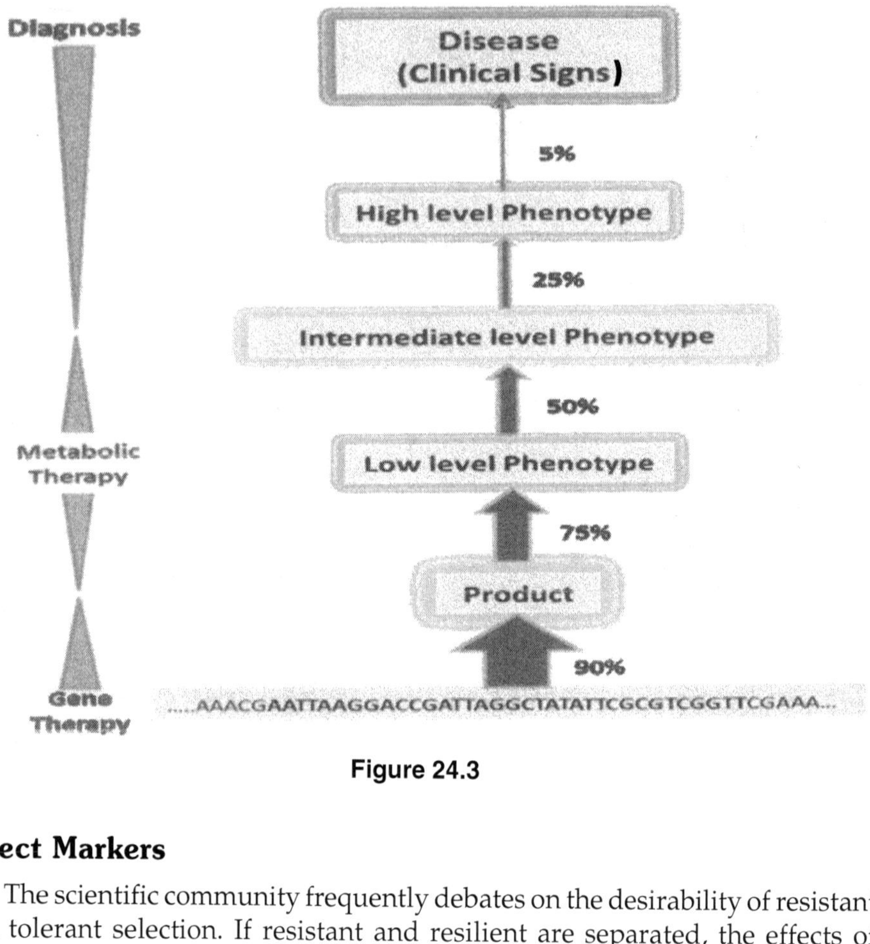

Figure 24.3

Direct Markers

The scientific community frequently debates on the desirability of resistant and tolerant selection. If resistant and resilient are separated, the effects of improving the two attributes could be very different. Improved resistance, should minimise infection transmission between animals, but improved tolerance will decreases the indication of clinical sickness but not necessarily infection transmission. Unselected animals added into the population would benefit from improved herd-level resistance in the former situation, whereas unselected animals in the same habitat would be at danger of disease in the latter case (Lewis *et al.*, 2007).

Genes that influence performance and those that control resistance are not linked. As a result, genetic correlation between resistance and performance can be viewed of as the result of a balance between two opposing factors: the host's immune response vs. infection (Goddard and Hayes, 2009). The association will be unfavourable if the resources used to defend the host outweigh the advantages of becoming more resistant. The relationship will be favourable if the benefits of being resistant, that is, the damage prevented, balance the costs of gaining resistance (Bishop, 2012).

This concept forecasts genotype-by-environment interactions; for example, animal performance rankings may varied in contexts with different levels of challenge. Baker *et al.*, 2004 demonstrated that the Red Maasai sheep breed show more resistance to nematode resistance in high nematode challenge compared to low nematode dose challenge.

Apart from Faecal egg counts (FEC), Bishop (2012) claims that several indicator features are taken into account when selecting for resistance, including: (i) resistance measures: FEC, worm burden, worm size, and fecundity; (ii) immune response measures: eosinophilia, and antibodies such as IgA, IgG, and IgM; (iii) infection impact measures: anaemia, gastrin, pepsinogen, or fructosamine concentrations; and (iv) resilience measures: growth rate and required treatment frequency. Although the worm and larval count provide an important basis for epidemiological studies, but they are tedious, time consuming thus limits their use for routine monitoring and diagnosis. Apart from worm count, serological and ELISA tests provides useful diagnostic tools for worm burden in livestock herd.

Indirect Markers

Despite its benefits, the FEC takes time to measure and may not represent all of the process involved in internal nematode resistance because of physiological complexity (Douch *et al.*, 1996). Increased levels of IgG, IgE, and IgM in Romney selection line sheep were shown to be adversely connected with FEC, however IgE was also found to be negatively correlated with breech soiling. IgA immunoglobulin, which is tightly linked to immunological responses in the gut mucosa, has also been linked to resistance (Douch *et al.*, 1996). IgA can prevent larvae from developing in the stomach by functioning as an antibody to a *T. colubriformis* L3 carbohydrate surface antigen (CarLA), resulting in fast evacuation (Shaw *et al.*, 2013).

An important concept is that other disease-control strategies also have an antagonistic effect on genetic resistance to disease, as they allow the use of otherwise unfit animals in the breeding population by limiting natural selection to disease.Animal diseases significantly reduce the profitability because the identification of the phenotype for disease resistance is difficult in early stage. All healthy animals in a population may not be disease-resistant. Subclinical infections can exist in animals that appear to be healthy. These could be thought of as pathogen reservoirs. It's also possible that the amount of exposure given to susceptible animals was insufficient to produce disease. The FAMACHA technique was developed to assist parasite control by target-specific therapy (Van Wyk and Bath, 2002), based on the association between the colour of the eye mucus and the haematocrit values (level of anaemia). The FAMACHA score, when supplemented with simple penalties, may allow for fast genetic analyses within flocks. These could give producers the ability to choose from a pool of candidate sires and dams based on ranked predicted breeding values for FAMACHA scores in order to improve internal parasite resistance and/ or resilience, with the ultimate goal of producing animals that can live and produce better under relatively severe internal parasite challenges. It can be used as a selection criterion if an animal survives and reproduces without being dewormed.

Differences between Breeds

For the FEC, genetic variations across and within breeds have been observed (McManus *et al.*, 2011). Most studies have reported that the locally adapted breeds are more resistant to disease compared to commercial breeds. This could be attributed to the low production of locally adapted breeds, which have a slower growth rate than commercial varieties. Because less demand is imposed on nutritional partition of elements that affect both growth and resilience, such as protein quantity in the feed, the lower genetic potential for growth has an impact on resilience. Locally adapted Morada Nova and Bergamasca had the lowest FEC for *Strongylide*, whereas locally adapted Santa Ines and its cross with Ile de France (Ile X SI) had the lowest values for *Strongyloides* (McManus *et al.*, 2011). On the other hand, Ile de France sheep had the lowest faecal oocyst count of *Eimeria* spp. In these sheep, there were few genetic associations between the FEC or FOC and parasite species, and heritability estimate range from 0.09 to 0.31.

A study in Kenya has reported that Red Maasai lambs had lower FECs for *Haemonchus contortus* and reduced mortality compared to Dorper lambs. Under these parasite-friendly subhumid environments of Kenya, the Red Maasai flocks were predicted to be two to three folds more prolific than the Dorper animals. Similarly, it has been discovered that Indonesian Thin-Tailed sheep are more resistant to disease than St. Croix and Merino sheep (Roberts *et al.*, 1997).

Selection and Crossbreeding may Affect Breed Resistance

The locally adapted Santa Ines of Brazil has been claimed as endoparasitic resistant breed. However, this has not been substantiated in other studies, generally in comparisons with commercial breeds (McManus *et al.*, 2011). Under mild *H. contortus* infection, Bricarello *et al.* (2005) reported no significant variations in haematological and biochemical profiles between Ile de France and Santa Ines lambs. Studies have revealed that when resistant and susceptible breeds are crossed, variation in degree of resistance of the crossbred progeny is observed. This variation in resistance depends on the breed, age of the animal, and whether the tests were conducted using natural or manufactured illnesses. Disease control can be aided by managing genetic resources in order to improve the resistance or resilience of cattle herds.

Selective breeding to exploit within-breed disease resistance variation is an essential method in the control of a number of illnesses. However, selection for resistane alone results in reduction of production trains such as decreased live weight,and fleece weight (Snowder, 2006). As a result, appropriate selection policies are required, but the main indirect benefit of resistance is reduced pasture pollution. Because there is no drop in FEC, non-resilient animals in the flock face a higher parasite burden from resilient animals, who are basically asymptomatic carriers. Bisset and Morris, 1996 has reported high genetic association (0.56) resistance and resilience as high as 0.56, and greater heritability estimates in resistance compared to resilience.

Host genetic resistance is assumed to be breaking down as nematodes evolve to adapt to resistant hosts. However, the evolution of parasites should be slower than parasitic resistance due to the polygenic nature of parasite resistance, as worms would have to evolve against a far larger number of targets (Bishop, 2012). Kemper *et al.* (2013) investigated three hypothesised mechanisms for the influence of sheep genotype on FEC in sheep: (i) decrease worm establishment, (ii) raise adult worm mortality, and (iii) decrease adult egg production. They discovered that because the genes only impact female worms and not the males, when sheep resistance reduces adult egg production, it puts less selective pressure on the worm population. As a result, when the resistance genes act on both sexes, the amount of the gain for resistant worms is just half of what it is when the resistance genes act on both sexes.

As a result, it is possible to test multiple evolutionary solutions to the same problem. According to Gibson and Bishop (2005), the following factors should be considered when deciding on genetic improvement priorities: There is sufficient genetic variation for disease resistance between or within breeds to allow effective genetic improvement; there are clear economic and social benefits due to genetic improvement of resistance, allowing for the use of other methods of disease control; there are clear economic and social benefits due to genetic improvement of resistance, allowing for the use of other methods of disease control (used as an alternative to, or in conjunction with, host resistance).Direct selection, where heredity is often medium to low, leads in slow selection for these traits, and economic values are generally modest (McManus *et al.*, 2014), but are heavily influenced by the cost of diagnosis and treatment.

Genotype X Environment Interaction

According to Castillo-Juarez *et al.* (2000) and Kearney *et al.* (2004), animals adapt to the environment in which they are selected, hence environmental sensitivity is unlikely to result from selection for enhanced production levels. Unfavourable genetic associations of milk yield with somatic cell score and conception rate were substantially higher in a poor environment than in a good environment.

McManus *et al.* (2014) reported that breeds react differently to different pasture types in terms of feed quality and availability, resulting in variable FEC findings. According to Scholtz *et al.* (2013), due to projected changes in habitats as a result of global warming and climate change, genotype-environment matching will be critical to ensuring a long-term rise in production. Optimal production systems are ones that are environmentally friendly and use the right genotypes, and they should be developed when they aren't already in existence. Thus, the sustainability of production system could be achieved when the changing environment is linked with the breeding strategies.

Genetic Markers

Locally adapted breeds must be integrated into current production systems in order to survive. In these breeds, significant features that may play an important role in specific market niches must be found. A wide range of technologies are being utilised to improve the identification of desirable features since the discovery of molecular techniques (Springbett *et al.*, 2003). However, Kemper *et al.* (2013) has reported that since the polymorphism used in marker assisted selection is dependent on within-family linkage. Thus, finding associations in the different population without polymorphic loci is difficult. The segregation of families on the basis of polymorphism is not possible due to fixation of polymorphic allele or low allele frequencies in that population. Because of differences in the linkage phase between families, reproducing linkage results by identifying multiple linked QTLs is especially problematic. For worm resistance, many researchers have inferred the coding region of interferon gamma (IFNG) gene in major histocompatibility complex (MHC).

When an animal is confronted by viruses or parasites, the MHC involves a series of highly polymorphic genes that are responsible for the activation of the immune response. The MHC is linked to a variety of animal production features, including sheep (Santucci *et al.*, 2007). Nematode resistance has been linked to QTLs on chromosomes 1, 2, 3, 6, 14, and 20 in several studies (Davies *et al.*, 2006). DRB1, OARCP73, DYMS1, and BM1815 are among the QTLs reported on chromosome 20. MHC markers (CP73, DYMS1), and FEC (BM1815) has been reported to be significantly associated with haematocrit (CP73), IgL (immunoglobulin lambda) level (DYMS1), and FEC (BM1815) in Roehnschaf flock artificially challenged with *H. contortus*. Non-*Nematodirus Strongyle* FEC has been linked to microsatellite markers on chromosome 20 in Scottish Blackface sheep (Davies *et al.*, 2006).

The search for quantitative trait loci (QTLs) for nematode resistance in animals is a tough task, due its physiological and behavioural complexity.Most studies based on low-resolution genome screens, results in extremely wide confidence ranges. These investigations varies according to the breeds, their immune condition, parasite species, level of resistance and challenge regimens of parasite. Given the complexity of nematode resistance, it's not unexpected that past research hasn't always produced the same results.

Genome-wide Selection

SNP (single nucleotide polymorphisms) is the variation of single nucleotide in the DNA sequence of homologous chromosome. These variations can occur in the whole genome including protein coding regions known and non-protein coding regions, such as regulatory regions. Changes in regulatory sequences are thought to have significant role in the evolution of morphology, physiology, and behaviour (Carroll, 2000). Recent studies have investigated the, availability and importance of a genome-wide set of SNPs has paved the way for more research in the area of disease resistance (McManus *et al.*, 2014). Moreover, several non-coding RNAs like micro RNAs and long non-coding RNAs also regulate the expression of gene at various level. Genome-wide association studies (GWAS) aims to uncover the genetic basis of prevalent diseases, have been implemented as a result of breakthroughs in genomics technology, statistical approaches and bioinformatics.

Conclusions

The complex process of immune system and parasitic infection reflect long period of host-parasite coevolution. The capacity to use diagnostic tests to detect the onset of anthelmintic resistance at an early stage is a crucial part of treating it. Diagnostics may play an essential role in determining which medications remain effective in host-parasite systems where resistance is already widespread. Genetic Variation in disease resistance between different breeds and species could suggest role of genetics in disease resistance. Selection of locally adapted breed in their environmental conditionis the first step, followed by phenotypic resistance selection. Adaptation to local environment and genotype-environment interaction may influence the genetic variation for resistance in livestock. Thus, selection indicesof animals should includedisease resistance as well as for performance trait together, as it is expected that the parasite willnot evolve quickly in response to resistant hosts. Our future researches should aim for selecting disease resistant animal to improve productivity of animal.

REFERENCES

Baker, R.L., Mugambi, J.M., Audho, J.O., Carles, A.B. and Thorpe, W. (2004). Genotype by environment interactions for productivity and resistance to gastro-intestinal nematode parasites in Red Maasai and Dorper sheep. *Animal Science*, **79:** 343–353.

Bishop, S.C. (2012). A consideration of resistance and tolerance for ruminant nematode infections. *Frontiers in Genetics*, **3**: 1–7.

Bishop, S.C. and Morris, C.A. (2007). Genetics of disease resistance in sheep and goats. *Small Ruminant Research*, **70**: 48–59.

Bisset, S.A., Morris, C.A. (1996). Feasibility and Implications of breeding sheep for resilience to nematode challenge. *International Journal for Parasitology*, **26**(8/9): 857–868.

Bricarello, P.A., Amarante, A.F.T., Rocha, R.A. (2005). Influence of dietary protein supply on resistance to experimental infections with Haemonchus contortus in Ile de France an Santa Inês lambs. *Veterinary Parasitology*, **134**(11): 99–109.

Carroll, S. (2000). Endless forms: the evolution of gene regulation and morphological diversity. *Cell*, **101**: 577–580.

Castillo-Juarez, H., Oltenacu, P.A., Blake, R.W., McCulloch, C.E. and Cienfuegos-Rivas, *e.g.* (2000). Effect of herd environment on the genetic and phenotypic relationships among milk yield, conception rate, and somatic cell score in Holstein cattle. *Journal of Dairy Science*, **83**: 807–814.

Cheng, H.H., Kaiser, P. and Lamont, S.J. (2013). Integrated genomic approaches to enhance genetic resistance in chickens. *Annual Review Animal Bioscience*, **1**: 239-260.

Davies, G., Stear, M.J., Benothman, M., Abuagob, O., Kerr, A., Mitchell, S. and Bishop, S.C. (2006). Quantitative trait loci associated with parasitic infection in Scottish Blackface sheep. *Heredity*, **96**: 252–258.

Douch, P.G.C., Green, R.S., Morris, C.A., McEwan, J.C. and Windon, R.G. (1996). Phenotypic markers for selection of nematode-resistant sheep. *International Journal for Parasitology*, **26**(8–9): 899–911.

Gibson, J.P. and Bishop, S.C. (2005). Use of molecular markers to enhance resistance of livestock to disease: a global approach. *International Office of Epizootics*, **24**(1): 343–353.

Goddard M. E. and Hayes B. J. (2009). Mapping genes for complex traits in domestic animals and their use in breeding programmes. *Nature Reviews Genetics*,**10**: 381–391.

Kearney, J.F., Wall, E., Villanueva, B., and Coffey, M.P. (2004). Inbreeding trends and application of optimized selection in the UK Holstein population. *Journal of Dairy Science*, **87**: 3503-3509.

Kemper, K.E., Goddard, M.E. and Bishop, S.C. (2013). Adaptation of gastrointestinal nematode parasites to host genotype: single locus simulation models. *Genetics Selection Evolution*, **45**(14): 1–14.

Lewis, C.R.G., Ait-Ali, T., Clapperton, M., Archibald, A.L. and Bishop, S. (2007). Genetic perspectives on host responses to porcine reproductive and respiratory syndrome (PRRS). *Viral Immunology*, **20**(3): 343–357.

McManus, C., Dallago, B.S.L., Louvandini, H., Melo, C.B., Seixas, L.S. and Oliveira, F.J.G. (2013). Gastrointestinal parasitism in sheep kept on Andropogon and Panicum pastures in the Federal District, Brazil. *Journal of Animal Science Advances*, **3**(5): 214–21

McManus, C., Louvandini, H. and Gugel, R. (2011). Skin and coat traits in sheep in Brazil and their relation with heat tolerance. *Tropical Animal Health and Production*, **43**: 121–126.

McManus, C., Paim, T.P., Barros de Melo, C., S. A. F. Brasil, C.S.A.F. and Paiva, S.R. (2014). Selection methods for resistance to and tolerance of helminths in livestock.*Parasite,* **21** (56): 1-15

Mueller, M. and Brem, G. (1994). Transgenic strategies to increase disease resistance in livestock. *Reproduction and Fertility Development,* **6**: 605-613.

Roberts, J.A, Estuningsih, E., Widjayanti, S., Wiedosari, E., Partoutomo, S. and Spithill, T.W. (1997). Resistance of Indonesian thin tail sheep against *Fasciola gigantica* and *F. hepatica. Veterinary Parasitology,* **68**(1–2): 69–78.

Santucci, F., Ibrahim, K.M. and Hewit, G.M. (2007). Selection on MHC-linked microsatellite loci in sheep populations. *Heredity,* **99**: 340–348.

Scholtz, M.M., Maiwashe, A., Neser, F.W.C., Theunissen, A., Olivier, W.J., Mokolobate, M.C. and Hendriks, J. (2013). Livestock breeding for sustainability to mitigate global warming, with the emphasis on developing countries. *South African Journal of Animal Science,* **43**(3): 269–281.

Shaw, R.J., Morris, C.A. and Wheeler, M. (2013). Genetic and phenotypic relationships between carbohydrate larval antigen (CarLA) IgA, parasite resistance and productivity in serial samples taken from lambs after weaning. *International Journal for Parasitology,* **43**(8): 661–667.

Snowder, G. (2006). Genetic selection for disease resistance: challenges and opportunities. *Beef Improvement Federation Conference Proceedings,* **38**: 52–60.

Springbett, A.J., MacKenzie, K., Woolliams, J.A. and Bishop, S.C. (2003). The contribution of genetic diversity to the spread of infectious diseases in livestock populations. *Genetics,* **165**(3): 1465–1474.

Van Wyk, J.A. and Bath, G.F. (2002). The FAMACHA system for managing haemonchosis in sheep and goats by clinically identifying individual animals for treatment. *Veterinary Research,* **33**: 509–529.

Index

B

C

D

E

F

G

H

I

K

L

M

N

O

P

Q

R

S